Partnership Working in Mental Health Care

For Anne and Philip

For Elsevier

Commissioning Editor Susan Young
Development Editor Catherine Jackson
Project Manager Wendy Gardiner / Morven Dean
Designer Judith Wright

Partnership Working in Mental Health Care

The Nursing Dimension

Keith Edwards PhD MA BA CertEd RMN RNT ILTM

Principal Lecturer in Mental Health Nursing, Buckinghamshire Chilterns University College, Buckinghamshire, UK

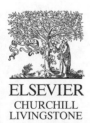

ELSEVIER
CHURCHILL
LIVINGSTONE

EDINBURGH LONDON NEW YORK OXFORD PHILADELPHIA ST LOUIS SYDNEY TORONTO 2005

ELSEVIER
CHURCHILL
LIVINGSTONE

First published 2005

ISBN 0 443 07397 X

British Library Cataloguing in Publication Data
A catalogue record for this book is available from the British Library

Library of Congress Cataloging in Publication Data
A catalog record for this book is available from the Library of Congress

Note
Knowledge and best practice in this field are constantly changing. As new
research and experience broaden our knowledge, changes in practice, treatment
and drug therapy may become necessary or appropriate. Readers are advised to
check the most current information provided (i) on procedures featured or (ii) by
the manufacturer of each product to be administered, to verify the recommended
dose or formula, the method and duration of administration, and
contraindications. It is the responsibility of the practitioner, relying on their own
experience and knowledge of the patient, to make diagnoses, to determine
dosages and the best treatment for each individual patient, and to take all
appropriate safety precautions. To the fullest extent of the law, neither the
publisher nor the author assumes any liability for any injury and/or damage.

The Publisher

 your source for books,
journals and multimedia
in the health sciences
www.elsevierhealth.com

The
publisher's
policy is to use
**paper manufactured
from sustainable forests**

Printed in China

Contents

Chapter 1

Introduction

INTRODUCTION

During the second half of the 20th century there has been growing criticism of mental health services and during the last two decades this criticism has resulted in extensive changes in the delivery of those services. Seeking out and listening to the views of those who use the services has become part of the strategy for change, but how far have those changes gone to ensure that users' voices are really being heard? In 1993, Davey reported that:

'Psychiatric users like myself have the persistent experience that staff, doctors and nurses do not listen to what we say. This is sometimes vehemently denied by people who do not know the difference between hearing and listening. Within the medical model what we say is not being listened to for its original meaning but for signs of pathology. What we say is not being listened to; it is being examined for evidence for the purpose of diagnoses.'

Ten years on, other service users describe their experiences likewise:

'I have problems telling my psychiatrist about the negative aspect of my daily life. This is because problems can mean an increase in medication or admission to the ward'. (Openmind 2001) and

> 'most psychiatrists and nurses, I feel, have little understanding of mental distress. Many are presumptuous and assume that if a person "looks all right" or "looks well" then they must be a malingerer. I have known at least fifteen people who "looked well" but have since committed suicide.' (Openmind 2002)

More and more user groups have emerged in response to the beliefs of the recipients of mental health services that their views were not sought or taken into consideration when services were being planned. As one user put it, 'the fact that one is a user is not sufficient grounds to exclude and invalidate the views of users as is often the case'(Campbell 1991). Thus it has been the past experience of users that their views were seldom sought. Rickets and Kirshbaum (1994) suggest that even when such views were sought they were seldom acted upon. It is clear that a considerable impetus for enquiry and criticism has come from the experiences and dissatisfaction of those who have been, and continue to be, users of mental health services. This in turn has been taken up by policy makers and incorporated into strategies for change. Hence, with the upsurge of user groups and the present climate of change it appears to be an opportune time for some of these developments to be reflected upon within the context of partnership in mental health care with users at the centre of developments and change.

The broad aim of this book is to examine the notion of partnership in care and to evaluate the role of mental health nursing in the context of meeting the needs of the users of mental health services. It seeks to determine the extent to which users perceive their needs as being met and, if not, to ascertain what changes are required regarding the preparation and the role of the mental health nurse as a key player in their care. The research for this book was considered within the context of the broader political climate of change within health service provisions and taking into account the various policy documents that have been published to improve the nature and quality of the health service (Department of Health 1992, 1997a, 1997b, 1998a, 1998b, 1998c, 1999a, 2001a, 2001b, Sainsbury Centre for Mental Health 1997). The intention is to contribute to an understanding of both a user and mental health nursing perspective in the context of partnership working in mental health care, in the hope that this can play a part in enhancing the quality of the service.

At the turn of the millennium the issue of user perspectives had been clearly placed on the mental health agenda. Prior to this period there was a paucity of literature regarding the views of users of mental health services and Raphael (1977), Campbell (1996), Rogers et al (1993) and Lovell (1995) argued that the possible reason for the lack of published literature and of research into this area was due to a widely held belief that the mental health status of users renders their viewpoint erroneous. Despite this, the late 1990s have seen an upturn in the amount of attention that is now being paid to eliciting such views. This indicates a paradigm shift that has taken place during that time, from considering users of mental health services as objects of care and treatment to considering them as participants and partners in their own care. Thus, the published literature has become more service user focused and there has been a corresponding shift in mental health policy. The research into aspects of care giving by mental health nurses from the perspective of those that use the services has become increasingly relevant and timely for mental health service provision. However, we need to be cautious about the research and evidence that has traditionally tended to dominate in the field of mental health. We need to reflect carefully on its validity, reliability and the extent to which it reflects the real voice and experience of those who use mental health services.

The climate for change calls for evidence-based practice but there appears to be a considerable gap between research and clinical practice. Geddes et al (1997) suggest that there are 'two explanations for this situation, either there is no evidence on which to base practice or that there is evidence but it is not being used and, as such, users are not receiving the best available care. One essential ingredient required to make mental health services clinically effective is to ensure that clinicians keep up to date and know how to use evidence. In addition to the problems of keeping up to date common to all clinicians, mental health practitioners are often geographically isolated from information resources'. The only time that many update their knowledge is when they attend a course of study rather than on a regular basis. Hopefully the notion and the promotion of life-long learning will help to change this cultural tradition.

Goding and Edwards (2002) suggest that, on the surface, the concept of evidence-based practice (EBP) is seductive, and that there should be no disagreement with practice being underpinned by evidence. There is, however, a danger that concepts such as EBP are promoted and taken on board without sufficient debate, dialogue and investigation of what is really involved. We would all probably agree with the intent of wanting to provide the best possible care, underpinned by the best available evidence, but we have to be careful whose research and evidence tends to dominate: is it valid and reliable? A hierarchy of evidence tends to prevail, with Randomised Controlled Trials (RCTs) being seen as the gold standard of research – but how appropriate are RCTs in certain complex human situations and environments? Are RCTs appropriate for complex, subjective conditions such as mental health and life choices in general? Geddes et al (1997) further indicate that 'the provision of mental health services is determined by many factors, including government policy, public demand, the behaviour of general practitioners and mental health professionals, and the financial pressures under which purchasers and providers of services work. These groups often have widely disparate views about the nature of mental disorder and the most appropriate services, and many forces exist to keep their views apart'. Hence no analysis of our present provision of mental health services would be complete, or a proper understanding achieved, without examining the historical, philosophical and political context.

Criticism of mental health services is not new and has typically come from those that provide the service. During the second half of the 20th century there was growing concern about the ideology and practice of institutional care. During the 1960s an anti-psychiatry movement was led by doctors who believed that the service provided was doing more harm than good and that the whole system of psychiatry needed a thorough overhaul (Cooper 1968, Laing & Esterson, 1964).Theorists such as Foucault (1967), Szasz (1971), Goffman (1961) and Scull (1997) have also been very powerful critics of the lack of effectiveness of psychiatry. Butler and Pritchard (1983) and Handyside and Heyman (1994) argue that mental illness is culturally specific and that a mental disorder is a social construct, thus questioning the medical foundation of psychiatry, which they perceive as failing to achieve effective outcomes. Bowers (1998) from a nursing perspective criticises the theories of mental illness as a social construct but concludes that, though sometimes misguided, they cannot be wholly rejected. Some people are turning away from conventional psychiatry for solutions to their mental health problems; for example there is a growing number of self-help, user-led groups and alternative therapies that challenge the dominance of a medical model of mental illness. Whatever the solutions offered by critics it has become clear that any consideration of mental health must take account of the environment in which individuals live their lives and that mono-causal explanations of mental illness are unconvincing.

The criticisms have reflected the changing world view within western thought. The ancient world was regarded as stable and controlled by religion and magic. Modern social theorists challenged that. They saw the modern world as progressive and dominated by rationality and a belief in the ultimate discovery of the scientific truth. Postmodernism embraces a range of movements and ideas that fundamentally confront those values and beliefs. Kelly and Chalton (1995) see postmodernism as 'the world of aesthetics, the deconstruction of conventional social arrangements and of experimentation in culture, art and life. It is a fundamental break with the past; life is viewed as chaotic and uncertain. Instead of progress there is change with reality being defined as paradoxical, ambiguous and open-ended'. Intrinsic within the change from modernism to postmodernism has been an undermining of institutions and the rise of the individual. Against this background many users of mental health services have found their voice, a voice that is increasingly demanding attention.

The last two decades have also been a time of profound change within the philosophy of the Welfare State, as it has been known since its post-war inception. Rationalisation, reforms and restructuring were high on the previous government's agenda and continue to be so under a Labour administration. In recent years, mental health policy has been overhauled in an attempt to create a system of care which can truly support people with mental health problems. There have been a number of publications produced by Government for change; for example, *Caring for People* (Department of Health 1989) was a significant White Paper reflecting some progressive thinking by suggesting that services should be designed to meet the needs of the individual and that a voice for users should be provided. It also suggested that carers should be supported and help provided for people with disabilities to lead an ordinary life in the community. Concern about continuity of health care has also been raised and it was suggested that there should be greater collaborative arrangements between health authorities and social services if a truly integrated system of care is to prevail. The National Health and Community Care Act (Department of Health 1990) went even further in recommending that the needs of users and carers must be considered in relation to service provision. Almost 10 years later *The National Health Service Plan* (1999b) set out to transform the health and social care system so that it would produce faster, fairer services that delivered better health care, and to tackle health inequalities. *The National Service Framework for Mental Health* (Department of Health 1999c) also identified seven standards to be achieved as part of the change process:

- Standard 1: Health and Social Services should promote mental health for all, combat discrimination and promote social inclusion.
- Standard 2: Users who contact their Primary Health Care team should have their needs assessed and identified and offered effective treatment.
- Standard 3: Users should be able to make contact with NHS Direct and be referred to local or specialist services 24 hours a day.
- Standard 4: All users of the Care Programme Approach should have a written and agreed care plan that is regularly reviewed and that anticipates or prevents a crisis, reduces risk and provides support 365 days a year.
- Standard 5: Care away from home should be as unrestrictive as possibly whilst protecting the individual and the public. There should be an identified care coordinator and the identification of what action to take in a crisis.
- Standard 6: There should be care for carers.
- Standard 7: Preventing suicide, the previous six standards to apply plus staff should be competent to assess risk.

Modernising Mental Health Services (Department of Health 2002) also set out to create safe, sound and supportive mental health services, through a variety of measures including the introduction of more intensive community support services such as 'assertive outreach teams' to address the problems of people living in the community with complex needs. It is certainly true that mental health is being giving a higher priority than ever before and with real growth in spending. This is a welcome development but at times the ideas for change have remained rhetorical and have not been translated into the reality of everyday care. It is the implementation of change that has been the most difficult aspect to achieve.

Current policy is emphatic that people should be cared for in their own environments and that the new welfare services should be based on certain choices and underpinned by various charter rights. This approach was formally expressed in *The Patient's Charter* (Department of Health 1991) which stated in its Foreword that 'the service should always put the patient first and be responsive to people's views and needs'. The approach contrasts with earlier philosophies of care that placed the user in a passive role, emphasising the removal of people from their domestic and social context. The draft *Patient's Charter – Mental Health Services* suggested that the National Health Service could learn from service users, encouraging feedback of their experience, be it good or bad, to propel improvements. *The Mental Health Services Patient's Charter* that was published in 1997 (Department of Health 1997a) then set out a number of new and improved standards for users. The main areas covered were effective discharge and aftercare arrangements and better information to enable people with mental health problems to get the services that they need. The Charter's emphasis on better information suggested 'information on issues of diagnosis; drugs and their effects; the availability of services and alternative treatments; what to do in an emergency and the provision of local advocacy and support groups. It was hoped that greater access to information would enable users and their carers to play a more informed part in their mental health care'.

In March 1998 the Government announced that it had become their official policy that there would be a new emphasis on patients' views in shaping the future of the National Health Service as well as a national annual survey of patients' experiences. (Department of Health 1998d) The Health Secretary, speaking at the opening ceremony of the International Symposium to celebrate the 50th Anniversary of the World Federation for Mental Health, also announced that 'tackling mental health issues will be one of the major challenges facing us in the 21st century and this work will call for partnership at all levels, between agencies, between individual countries, users of mental health services and policy makers' (Department of Health 1998e).

This new direction in policy reflects the age of the pre-eminence of the rights of the individual. Empowerment has become the buzzword for many areas of human activity. Within mental health 'service users' are replacing 'patients', passive recipients of care. These users are to become more involved in the services they use by being alerted to the resources within themselves and within their communities. The rise of individual rights also brings with it responsibility for oneself. Responsibility for one's welfare and journey through life is now removed from formally paternalistic institutions and located within individuals. More influence and control on the part of mental health service users suggests an encroachment on the monopoly and control previously enjoyed by those that provided the service, the professionals, who were considered to know best and hence identified the needs of service users. It is unclear whether current policies aim fundamentally to empower users or to disempower professions. However, the goal is to create a service that meets users' needs and professionals may have to accept the implications of that for the traditional power relationships.

Charters started as a way of expressing the aspirations of users and have been a mechanism through which users were able to influence the service agenda; guides to the NHS have now replaced them. However, the extent to which charters could result in a more profound recasting of culture and power relationships, from which emerges a more appropriate choice of services, is debatable. There is a difference between charters produced for people and charters produced by people; the former can be conceived as being someone else's agenda that is being imposed while a charter produced by the people via consultation and participation can be more representative. Hogg (1994) suggested that the agenda had already been taken over by government and managers. Furthermore, Mandelstam and Schwehr (1995) remind us that the exact legal status of such charter rights is difficult to ascertain and from a legal perspective charters are merely directional in nature. The policy of introducing charters may have served a political or economic purpose for government in presenting a popular measure to extend the rights of the individual in relation to monolithic public institutions but some scepticism may be justified as to the degree to which empowerment for service users has been extended and whether there will be any lasting effect.

Certainly some shift in power to service users has occurred, and this can be observed in language. Terminology such as user, client, stakeholder, customer and citizen has been introduced into our everyday speech, topical literature and policy documents. Although there does not appear to be any evidence that the term 'user' is liked or used by the majority of those people receiving mental health care, it is a word that appears to be in the ascendancy and is used as a way of moving the focus of attention to service users. However, the pressure to conform to the growing orthodoxy around the use of new language might result in mere 'lip service' to the words, a convenient way to soften medical language. A letter in *Openmind* Nov/Dec 1996 posed the question 'Do trendy synonyms do anything to challenge the basis of prejudice and stigma?' It further suggests, 'as long as people are marginalized and devalued, whether we call people 'users' or 'gold dust' the label will eventually become tarnished'. This kind of thinking indicates the relative powerlessness that some users may feel. Nevertheless, the power of semantics should not be underestimated and may have a profound effect in undermining previous models of welfare provision. Changes may move much further than policy makers initially intended. The real extent of the actual involvement and empowerment of users remains to be seen and will only become clearer as the reforms of state welfare unfold.

A great impetus for changing power relationships within mental health provision was the closure of the large Victorian psychiatric institutions, which gathered momentum in the 1990s and has been a major part of the reforms of state welfare from that time. Grove (1994) maintained that implicit in the movement towards community care was a shift in power between mental health workers and service users, resulting in more power for the user. However, as change towards community care proceeded, the pressure from forces of reaction has to a certain extent resulted in 'old wine in new bottles' – especially given a climate of fear arising from a badly informed population about restructured services and service users that are no longer 'out of sight'. Jones (1982) refers to the 'Scull dilemma' that confronts someone simultaneously critical of traditional mental hospitals and of so-called community care. Scull (1996) suggests that it is not his dilemma but society at large, since 'history presents us with inadequate, often inhumane and always under funded mental hospitals or a grossly underdeveloped and frequently non-existent system of community care'. This is a situation for which we all have to take some responsibility.

Such structural change has of course meant that the service also requires a new breed of mental health workers, professionals who can meet the challenges of the new system of service provision and relationship with service users. Previous nurse training produced nurses who often separated themselves from service users by their language, uniforms, titles and attitudes and closely followed the medical model of practice that tended to promote an aloofness from emotional issues (Menzies-Lyth 1970). As Pirsig (1974) observed, care 'happens when we are not separated from what we are working on, it involves a feeling of identification with what one is doing, to hurry something often indicates that you no longer care about it and want to get on to other things'.

Thus, nursing and nurse education is also undergoing fundamental change that is endeavouring to reorganise nursing in a similar way to other traditional professions. The works of Porter (1991) and Nolan (1993) show that the historical development of mental health nursing has a very weak training and knowledge base. Despite mental health nurses constituting the major human resource for mental health services, very few financial resources or opportunities have been made available to harness their real potential. Little attention was paid to the content of training; the assumption being that nurses would absorb additional information and good practice on the wards. Significantly, the confusion over what constituted good training only reflected the confusion that existed about what was good clinical practice. Looking back to the accommodation of mental health services into the National Health Service in 1948, little account had been taken of training needs as the early efforts of the newly formed NHS were focused on the acute (medical) sector and not on psychiatry. It is not surprising, therefore, that nurse training programmes had no history of taking into account user perspectives or actively involving users in some kind of partnership in the caring process. Eventually, *The Syllabus of Training 1982* (English and Welsh National Boards for Nursing, Midwifery and Health Visiting 1987) for Registered Mental Health Nurses incorporated within it 'client centeredness as a key principle' but its implementation has been somewhat slow.

At last, however, with the changes that are also taking place in nurse preparation, user perspectives have now been clearly put on the agenda. No current health and social policy document on mental health fails to mention the need to take user views into account or to involve them within service developments and provision. The introduction of *Project 2000* (United Kingdom Central Council for Nursing, Midwifery and Health Visiting 1986) has changed the base line of initial registration from certificate level to diploma and degree level. Schools of Nursing that were attached to hospitals have become integrated into higher education via universities. The integration into the university sector represents a considerable structural change for nurse education with the pressures to adapt to the structure and culture of universities. In some instances Schools of Nursing have established links with universities becoming Faculties of Health Studies and/or Schools of Health Sciences but have remained sited within their traditional settings. The linguistic shift from 'patient' to 'user' is mirrored by the titles of these nursing institutions that promote nursing as a science and an academic activity. However, the degree of real academic integration is questionable, particularly in the case of those facilities that have remained on their original site, which may result in a change in nursing culture coming about much more slowly. Interestingly, there are now moves afoot to move nurse education back to hospital environments in an attempt to develop a sense of identity and belonging with the hospital and to encourage employment and retention of staff. There is also debate about whether improved practice can be brought about by education alone and by modifying the nursing curriculum. Nolan (1993) points out that this belief has proved mistaken in the past and that lasting changes can only come about as a result of commitment at all levels of an organisation.

The changes that took place in the 1990s in pre-registration nurse education introduced three-year diploma and degree level courses that had a shared common foundation programme for the first 18 months and then a further 18 months specialisation in a branch programme (Mental Health, Learning Disabilities, Adult and Child). The hope was to be able to produce nurses who were more mature, confident and can accept responsibility, think analytically and flexibly and be prepared to develop professionally. The United Kingdom Central Council (1986) had the following hopes for nurse preparation when nurse education moved away from Schools of Nursing and into the higher educational sector:

- To win for nursing students the status and educational opportunities of other professional groups undertaking a vocational education;
- To terminate the practice of immersing students in hospital culture and ward routine;
- To establish links with institutes of Higher Education so that nursing education will receive academic validation;
- To improve morale in the profession so that recruitment of the 30,000 new nurses required each year in the UK might be assured (bearing in mind the reduced numbers of young people coming onto the job market) and their services retained;
- To place greater emphasis on health promotion and disease prevention than hitherto.

The above does not state specifically how users' views would relate to the role of the 'new nurse' but the implications are that a 'thinking and analytical' nurse would be able to be more responsive to the needs of users. Initial evaluation concerning the preparation of mental health nursing as reported by the *Working in Partnership* review team in 1994 revealed that there was 'widespread concern that the new programme (pre-registration) is not enabling students to develop sufficiently the essential skills of Mental Health Nursing' (Department of Health 1994). The report recommended (Recommendation 31) that 'the Statutory Bodies review the balance of time and emphasis given to each of the four branch programmes within the Common Foundation Programme' (Department of Health 1994).

In response to this the, English National Board for Nursing, Health Visiting and Midwifery (1995) issued revised criteria and guidelines for pre-registration nursing programme curriculum planners to:

- Ensure equity of both time and focus for each of the four branches of nursing within the Common Foundation Programmes.
- Review their teaching strategies to ensure that those providing input to the Common Foundation Programme are able to help students to set their learning within a mental health context.
- Ensure that there is articulation between the Common Foundation Programme and the Mental Health Branch Programme and that the developments of skills of the mental health nurse commence at the outset of the programme.

The English National Board for Nursing, Health Visiting and Midwifery (ENB) suggested the continual monitoring of these issues through the work of ENB officers and hoped that the needs of users would remain paramount as, with any agenda for change, vested interests in the status quo can easily come into play. The ENB has since become defunct and its role transferred to the Nursing and Midwifery Council (NMC) that has replaced the United Kingdom Central Council for Nursing, Midwifery and Health Visiting (UKCC).

The agenda for change in nurse education was primarily a way of increasing nursing confidence by offering nurses a higher education and thus a means of strengthening professional standing and improving salaries. It would be naive to consider that a user perspective was the key focus of that change. There is, however, a need for a true partnership with users of mental health services and a need to re-educate professionals in a way that takes cognisance of a user perspective. It may be too soon to evaluate with certainty whether or not recent and future generations of mental health nurses, having been exposed to a higher education programme, will make any significant change to how mental health or illness is viewed and practised. However, we do need to be able to answer the question of whether nurses have been prepared to meet the needs of service users from a user perspective and to what extent users' views, or their participation, have contributed to students' training and education and hence service provision and satisfaction. Research for this book looked at whether individual nurses, educated and trained under the new ethos of higher education, exhibit perceptions and prejudices which are receptive to the views and needs of users; to discover users' perception of mental health nursing; and in the light of the findings, to consider changes to the role of mental health nurses. For this purpose user views were sought and compared with the views of mental health nurses. The nursing sample consisted of those currently undertaking a nursing course as they were the most representative of mental health nurses being prepared under the most recent training scheme. The purpose was to endeavour to establish whether a new breed of nurse is being prepared to meet user needs within the context of the views of those that use mental health services.

The old order within mental health services, characterised by hierarchies, authority structures, promotional cultures and the concept that length of service constitutes a reason for conferring 'expertise' on individuals, has broken down. Seeking collaboration and partnership with users is but one expression of the new emerging order. The rise of a mental health user movement can be better understood within a post-modern context whereby users of the service are endeavouring to deconstruct the so-called scientific knowledge of medicine and are challenging the very power base of psychiatry. Those that use mental health services are clearly contributing their perspectives to the health care agenda and it would be foolish to ignore their perception of their reality. In the tradition of humanistic psychology Atkinson et al (1990) remind us 'humans must be understood in terms of their own subjective view of the world, the perception of self and their feelings of self worth'.

The expressed thoughts, feelings and experiences of users must be ascertained and taken seriously in the education and training of mental health nurses. Similarly, the role of mental health nurses must be clarified in terms of their self-perception, practice and the degree to which it meets the needs of those that use the services. The similarities and differences between a nursing and user perspective must be absorbed and acted upon within the provision of services, thus promoting identifiable competent practice that is clearly underpinned by the best available evidence.

References

Atkinson R L, Atkinson R C, Smith E E, Bem D J 1990 Introduction to psychology, 10th edn. Harcourt Brace Jovanovich, San Diego

Bowers L 1998 The social nature of mental illness. Routledge, London

Butler A, Pritchard C 1983 Social work and mental illness. Macmillan, Basingstoke

Campbell P 1991 We're not mad, we're angry (video). Mental Health Media, London

Campbell P 1996 Working with service users. In: Sandford T, Gournay K (eds) Perspectives in mental health nursing. Bailliere Tindall, London

Cooper D 1968 Psychiatry and anti-psychiatry. Tavistock, London

Davey B 1993 A user's view of psychiatric nursing - part II. The Journal of Mental Health Nursing Winter:10-14

Department of Health 1989 Caring for people. HMSO, London

Department of Health 1990 The National Health Service and Community Care Act: a brief guide. HMSO, London

Department of Health 1991 The patients charter. HMSO, London

Department of Health 1992 The health of the nation. The Stationary Office, London

Department of Health 1994 Working in partnership - report of the mental health nursing review team. HMSO, London, p 41

Department of Health 1997a The mental health services patients charter. HMSO, London

Department of Health 1997b Developing partnerships in mental health. HMSO, London

Department of Health 1998a Our healthier nation. The

Stationary Office, London

Department of Health 1998b Modernising mental health services - safe, sound and supportive. The Stationary Office, London

Department of Health 1998c The NHS plan. HMSO, London

Department of Health 1998d Press release 9th March 1998/084 Patients must be given greater say in the NHS - Milburn. Online. Available: http://www.coi.gov.uk/coi/depts/GDH/coi8699d.ok

Department of Health 1998e Press release 22nd October 1998/0448 International mental health symposium opens. Online. Available: http://www.coi.gov.uk/coi/depts/GDH/coi7062e.ok

Department of Health 1999a The national service framework. HMSO, London

Department of Health 1999b The national health plan. Department of Health, London

Department of Health 1999c The National Health Service framework for mental health. Department of Health, London

Department of Health 2001a The mental health policy implementation guide. HMSO, London

Department of Health 2001b Shifting the balance of power. HMSO, London

Department of Health 2002 Modernising mental health services. Department of Health, London

English and Welsh National Boards for Nursing, Midwifery and Health Visiting 1987 Syllabus of training 1982. EWNB, London

English and Welsh National Boards for Nursing, Midwifery and Health Visiting 1995 The Boards response to working in partnership. EWNB, London

Foucault M 1967 Madness and civilisation. Tavistock, London

Geddes J, Reynolds S, Streiner D, Szatmari P 1997 Evidence based practice in mental health. British Medical Journal 315(7121):1483-1484

Goding L, Edwards K 2002 Evidence based practice. Nurse Researcher 9(4):45-47

Goffman E 1961 Asylums. Penguin, Harmondsworth

Grove B 1994 Reform of mental health care in Europe: progress and change in the last decade. British Journal of Psychiatry 165:431-433

Handyside E, Heyman B 1994 Mental illness in the community: the role of voluntary and state agencies. In:

Heyman B (ed) Researching user perspectives on community health care. Chapman and Hall, London

Hogg C 1994 Beyond the patient's charter: working with users. Health Rights, London

Jones K 1982 Scull's dilemma. British Journal of Psychiatry 141:221-226

Kelly M P, Chalton B 1995 The modern and post-modern in health promotion. In: Bunton R, Nettleton S, Burrows R (eds) The sociology of health promotion. Routledge, London

Laing R D, Esterson A 1964 Madness and the family. Penguin, Harmondsworth

Lovell K 1995 User satisfaction with in-patient mental health services. Journal of Psychiatric and Mental Health Nursing 2(3):143-1484

Mandelstam M, Schwehr B 1995 Community care practice and the law. JKP, London

Menzies-Lyth I 1970 The functioning of social systems as a defence against anxiety in the community. Reprinted as Tavistock pamphlet no. 3. The Tavistock Institute of Human Relations, London

Nolan P 1993 History of mental health nursing. Chapman and Hall, London

Openmind, 112, Nov/Dec 2001;29

Openmind, 114, Mar/Apr 2002;25

Pirsig R M 1974 Zen and the art of motorcycle maintenance. Vintage, London

Porter R 1991 The Faber book of madness. Faber and Faber, London

Raphael W 1977 Psychiatric hospitals viewed by their patients. Kings Fund, London

Rickets T, Kirshbaum M N 1994 Helpfullness of mental health day care: client and staff views. Journal of Advanced Nursing 20:297-306

Rogers A, Pilgrim D, Lacey R 1993 Experiencing psychiatry: users' views of services. Macmillan/MIND, London

Sainsbury Centre for Mental Health 1997 Pulling together. The Sainsbury Centre for Mental Health, London

Scull A 1996 Asylums: utopias and realities. In: Tomlinson D, Carrier J (eds) Asylum and the community. Routledge, London, ch 15

Scull A 1997 Decaceration. Prentice-Hall, New Jersey

Szasz T 1971 The manufacture of madness. RKP, London

United Kingdom Central Council for Nursing, Midwifery and Health Visiting 1986 Project 2000: a new preparation for practice. UKCC, London

Chapter 2

Historical developments – nursing

CHAPTER CONTENTS

INTRODUCTION

History is an enquiry into the past that helps us to orientate ourselves to the here and now and to gain a sense of where we are going. It can be understood in the context of someone who has lost their memory: to enable them to discover who they are, they need to be conversant with their historical roots and developments and to be able to achieve this a reflection on the past is essential. Nolan's (1993 p124) book provides an excellent coverage of the roots of mental health nursing dating back to the 17th century. This chapter has no such ambition other than to focus on the period from the 1960s. The many reports and reviews emanating from government as well as published literature from professionals within the service and other academic writers about mental health nursing will be reflected upon.

In 1961 Enoch Powell, the Minister for Health at the time, made a speech indicating that the number of mentally ill patients was falling and that some of the large psychiatric hospitals belonged to a bygone age (Murphy 1991 p59, Nolan 1993 p126). In the following year the Ministry of Health (1962) launched its *Hospital Plan* that was the beginning of the official closure programme. Short stay psychiatric units attached to general hospitals and a greater focus upon community care would replace the large Victorian psychiatric hospitals. It followed that the role of the nurse also needed to change in response to these developments.

Over thirty years have elapsed since the publication of the review of mental health nursing in 1968 entitled *Psychiatric Nursing Today and Tomorrow* (Ministry of Health/Central Health Services council 1968). It was regarded, in its day, as a report that would make a significant contribution to the practice of psychiatric nursing. In 1994 we saw the arrival of another review of mental health nursing, *Working in Partnership – A Collaborative Approach to Care* (Department of Health 1994) that made recommendations for the way in which mental health nursing should develop. The following is a reflection on both these reports as well as the literature published during the interim period. An attempt will be made to ascertain to what degree mental health nursing has moved on from the publication of the 1968 and the 1994 reviews to the present day and to what extent the recommendations of both reports reflected the views of service users.

1968 – AGENDA FOR CHANGE

The terms of reference for the 1968 review were, 'To consider the functions of psychiatric nursing staff and, having regard to the changing pattern of psychiatric treatment, to make recommendations, firstly on nursing staff patterns in wards and departments of hospitals for the mentally ill and psychiatric units in general hospitals'.(Ministry of Health 1968 p1) The report only focused on hospital nursing and it seemed to espouse hospital care and a medical model approach; it had little to say about community nursing. On the initial page of the 1968 review it is noteworthy that those who expressed their views were mainly psychiatrists and the role of the nurse was seen to be moulded by the changing pattern of psychiatry. Ironically, the report acknowledges that 'it is not uncommon for medical staff to treat the nursing staff, even an experienced charge nurse, as an unskilled auxiliary whose views were of no account' (Ministry of Health 1968 p41).

In endeavouring to describe the function of the nurse, the 1968 review is somewhat equivocal. It refers to 'psychiatric nurses having round the clock responsibility for the care, comfort and well being of mentally ill people', and 'the nurse is therefore adaptable and versatile, ready, for example, to encourage and to organise patients' activities in such diverse fields as sport, music, millinery, camping or car maintenance'. Furthermore it suggests that, 'the essence of the nurse–patient relationship is that it arises mainly out of the events of life, some intimate, some casual, mostly spontaneous' (Ministry of Health 1968 pp14–15). Thus a clear emphasis was placed on nurses forming a therapeutic relationship with users rather than adopting a custodial approach to care. The report also suggested that initially relationships are intuitive but with training, insight develops and they are always (*sic*) able to make allowances for cultural differences of race, class and individual idiosyncrasies. Equally, by engaging with relatives of the patient, insight into their background and possible causes of their illnesses could be gained. It appeared that the report was attempting to define the important aspects of care, which British psychiatric nursing had failed to do, and it may well have provided the impetus for the studies of Altschul (1972 p11) and Cormack (1976) that examined the interactions between the nurse and the patient. Other factors that the report mentioned as being of significance for the psychiatric nurse were:

- Listening and counselling skills
- Basic nursing, for example patients' personal hygiene
- Observation
- Clear communication and administrative duties
- Nursing routine (that is, the organisation of the patient's day)
- Tasks and responsibilities clearly defined (e.g. the availability of check lists)
- All nurses should know patients in their wards as individuals, their names and their behaviour
- Maintaining ward supplies
- Physical and psychological treatments
- Continuity of patient care. On this issue the following was stated: 'We are concerned at the tendency in some hospitals to move staff more frequently than necessity dictates. This hinders developing relationships, tends to foster regimentalised uniformity and strongly hampers the development of good teamwork. We were shocked to hear of a hospital where all the staff nurses were re-assigned to different wards on 'moving day' – an arrangement that must destroy the development of any relationships between patients and nursing staff' (Ministry of Health 1968 p36).

Although concern was expressed about how teams work, it was suggested that, 'When in the care of a task-specified, differentiated group of professional staff organised on an authoritarian model, patients do badly; they are initially violent and ultimately subside into institutional apathy. When looked after by a good team, the patients retain or develop humanity, spontaneity and warmth and make progress towards recovery' (Ministry of Health 1968 p23).

The function of a ward was supposed to be determined by the requirements of the patients. Nurses would be required to provide physical nursing plus attention to personal needs such as hygiene, dressing and undressing and staff should show plenty of initiative, drive and experience. Attention was also drawn to the fact that insufficient nursing staff can do no more than the bare essentials of care and that over-pressed staff may slip into habits of carelessness, thoughtlessness and even callousness (Ministry of Health 1968 p40). On the other hand, the report suggested that nurses must be prepared to play a more advanced therapeutic role such as in the provision of group and behavioural therapy and at the same time be prepared for an increase in bedside nursing with the rising number of elderly patients. It was recognised that there was a need to appoint more domestic or clerical staff to relieve psychiatric nurses of non-nursing duties. In summary the 1968 review recommended:

- That there should be a more general study of domiciliary nursing of the mentally ill, including the roles of the psychiatric nurse, the public health nurse (i.e. the district nurse and the health visitor) and the social worker.

- That there should be further study of good administrative practice in psychiatric nursing in psychiatric hospitals and units.
- That there should be research into the personal or psychotherapeutic role of the nurse.
- That there should be a study of the problem of relieving nurses in psychiatric hospitals of non-nursing duties.
- That there should be studies aimed at identifying standards of nursing care and the associated staffing patterns with the object of trying to detect patterns of good practice that could be publicised regionally or nationally.

It appears that these recommendations were an attempt to redefine priorities whereby mental health nursing would be de-domesticated, making it less of a service to institutional maintenance and more of a service to patients.

Inquiries into failures in the system

Around the time that the 1968 review was published, vivid failures in the system began to emerge. Martin (1984) refers to the late 1960s and the 1970s as a period that saw a series of major scandals within the health service with at least ten inquiries of national significance and a whole string of lesser ones involving local inquiries. The issues of concern related to the failure of caring within hospitals, the misuse of drugs, shoddy conditions, neglect, fraud, maladministration and cruelty to patients. Martin considered that central to those failures was that, fundamentally, the quality of care came down to how individual staff members behaved to those in their care, 'that is the point where their skills, their human sympathy and their moral calibre are finally put to the test' (Martin 1984 pii). Following from that, the question was, what skills did these nurses have? Was it the case that they did not have the proper skills or that their skills were not attuned to the changing perception of how patients should be treated and the role that nurses were to fulfil? The nurse in the large institution was required to be proficient in practices of containment and control and according to Goffman (1961) they themselves were products of that system.

The culture that many of these inquiries identified during the 1970s was one not merely of allegations of violence, mistreatment of patients and lax over-administration of drugs but also one of a reluctance of staff to give evidence, reluctance to report bad incidents and hostility to those whom they called informers. A common thread that appears to emerge from all of these inquiries is the obstinate protection of the status quo by the nursing administration. In some of the hospitals Martin (1984 p13) reported that, 'an entrenched group of senior nurses succeeded for several years in suppressing the efforts by student nurses to do something about the ill treatment of patients on the wards. In essence over a period of four years student nurses had been complaining about the treatment of patients but very little was done to remedy the situation'. He further suggested that many of these inquiries were into problems stemming from a lack of new thinking and the dangers of corruption in closed societies, highlighted by the lengths to which staff and management would go to stifle criticism of the quality of care. Poor management and leadership were also cited as culpable. However, Martin also considered that the problems resulted from past inadequacies of provision,: hospitals were starved of resources, ensuring that trouble was unavoidable. It seems that this period depicts hospitals struggling to emerge from an era of prolonged deprivation and Martin concludes that from the literature of the day, the criticism of prolonged deprivation could easily be directed at mental health services generally.

The issues revealed by these inquiries are a reflection of the historical culture within mental health nursing and indicate the difficulties that are involved in initiating change. Such inquiries sadly continue to take place. Ashford Hospital in the 1990s has been investigated over allegations of drug and alcohol misuse, financial irregularities and possible paedophile activities. An inquiry led by Peter Fallon QC commenced in August 1997 (Department of Health 1997) and a report of its findings, published in 1999 (Department of Health 1999a), substantiated many of the allegations. It was the second major inquiry that the hospital had faced during the 1990s, with the first finding evidence of patients being 'systematically abused by staff, many of whom were nurses' (McMillan 1997). However, one has to be careful in drawing comparisons between the Special Hospitals and ordinary psychiatric hospitals as the history and culture differ significantly. Nevertheless, it is evidence that neglect and poor management still persists and this may support Martin's claim that neglect had become institutionalised within the culture of psychiatric nursing.

The changes of the 1980s

The 1968 review was explicit in placing the need for change on the agenda. This change acknowledged a move from 'patient' to 'service user' with whom those who work in mental health services must seek to form a partnership relationship as part of therapeutic forms of treatment. However, actual change was slow to come about and it was not until the 1980s that the agenda for change began to be put into practice. The motivation for the change emanated from economics and the perceived requirement to rationalise and cut back on expenditure. The 1980s have to be appreciated within the context of a society with high rates of unemployment, a very weak economic base and reluctance on the part of Government to increase funding to the public sector. Concern over the lack of resources during the 1970s heightened in the 1980s. The Conservative Government envisaged major structural changes and aimed to introduce market forces that they believed would make the NHS more accountable and give better value for money. The programme of hospital closure and the reduction of the numbers within the large Victorian institutions gathered momentum. This was promoted as a progressive development towards community care but it was also a money saving initiative. Community care was to be a partnership between families, the voluntary sector, the independent sector and the statutory services. In reflecting upon how that policy worked out in practice during the next decade, Zito and Howlett (1996) described it as 'neglect within the community and a burden imposed upon those least able to provide the necessary care and support'. They suggested that the infrastructure for effective community care was simply not in place and it is also possible that a culture of neglect has been relocated from psychiatric institutions into the community.

The changes in the 1980s brought with them a focus on nurse training and education in order to increase the awareness of nurses and for them to fulfil a new role. The 1982 syllabus of nurse training introduced changes to their preparation by incorporating many new initiatives that had not hitherto been addressed in training. It was designed to educate, not merely train, nurses, and to help them to develop skills that could be used both in the community and hospital settings. Much emphasis was given to interpersonal skills, the need for self-awareness, therapeutic relationships and to develop psychiatric nursing as a skilled profession. However the student nurses would depend for their training and practical clinical experiences on qualified nurses who were already well enmeshed into the existing culture. Nursing had been at the centre of the psychiatric culture within institutional settings and therefore, there was a danger of community care becoming a microcosm of the culture that was practised in the large psychiatric institutions (Ferguson & Brooker 1996, Nolan 1993). There appeared to be very little concern as to whether the clinical role models to which students were exposed would have a profound effect upon how the culture and practices within nursing developed and how change proceeded.

THE 1994 REVIEW

Following the extensive changes occurring during the 1980s, by the beginning of the 1990s it was felt that it was time to take stock of mental health nursing since there had not been a major review since 1968. The government announced in 1992 that it was to review mental health nursing in terms of its practice, education, research and management. The review was completed in 1994 and the terms of reference were, 'To identify the future requirements for skilled nursing care in light of developments in the provision of services for people with mental illness' (Department of Health 1994 piv). Virginia Bottomley, then Secretary of State for Health, in the Foreword of the report suggested that 'mental health nurses have a key role in ensuring that patients receive a high quality service in this challenging new era' (Department of Health 1994 pi). The hallmark of such a service would be characterised by a collaborative approach to care that met the needs of the individual. Equally, collaboration and partnership were also envisaged between other health care providers, professionals and carers. The review called for mental health nurses to be properly equipped with the skills to play their part in ensuring a quality service and to be able to move confidently between hospital and community settings. This had also been an aim of the 1982 syllabus of training. Within the context of the review it was also acknowledged 'that mental health nursing had not always been successful in providing good quality services that responded to people in their care' (Department of Health 1994 p9). In response to the above-mentioned issues the main body of the report made 42 recommendations under 6 themes:

1. *Expectations of mental health nurses*: This theme commences from the premise that 'it is a fundamental right that people who use mental health services can expect to receive skilled, sensitive, professional support from competent mental health nurses', a view that not many nurses would dispute. The review acknowledged that there had been a number of inquiries into neglect and mistreatment of long stay hospital residents during the 1960s and 1970s that had found belief in the above premise to be lacking (Department of Health 1994 p12). More positively, the review referred to a study by Rogers et al (1993 p42) into inpatient care which shows that 59% (n=280) of participants were either satisfied or very satisfied with the nursing care that they received, but that still left a large number who presumably were not satisfied with their care and treatment. The review also found that there was a need to ensure that nurses are more racially and culturally aware as people from black and other ethnic minority groups were treated differently, often shown less understanding and in the case of young black Afro-Caribbean men, more likely to be given a diagnosis of schizophrenia and admitted under a section of the Mental Health Act (Department of Health 1994 p12). The review furthermore addressed the need for appropriate information, treatment options and rights to be given to both users and carers. Other issues identified included the need to respect the wishes of the individual in relation to treatment, upholding dignity, users to be more involved in care planning and access to advocates. The need for appropriate staffing levels and skill mix was also recognised.

2. *The practice of mental health nurses*: The review was greatly concerned about the 'proper focus' of the mental health nurse and stated that those individuals in greatest need were not always targeted, especially those with a diagnosis of schizophrenia. Therefore, it recommended that the essential focus of the mental health nurse should be towards those with a 'serious or enduring mental illness'. That however begged the question, what is a non-serious mental illness? With regard to specific skills the review listed four pages of mutables under the heading of 'nursing skills' as articulated by the English National Board for Nursing but acknowledged that these are not exclusive to nurses. They were arranged in the format of the nursing process that sets out to offer a framework in which to assess, plan, implement and evaluate care. The nursing process was a step forward in that it offered a framework within which to begin to identify needs and hence to become aware of the possible skills required to meet those needs. The primacy of the individual and a more user-focused perspective were promoted and Recommendation 8 clearly called for the involvement of the individual in care planning and to take cognisance of their expressed wishes and needs.

Another key issue acknowledged by the review was skilled supervision and the need for this to become the norm within mental health nursing practice. The 1994 review considered that the 'therapeutic use of self' was at the core of mental health nursing and that it was essential that support and the opportunity for reflection and dialogue was made available to those responsible for providing the service.

3. *Mental health nurses and service delivery*: The review expressed concern regarding standards of management, lack of effective leadership and the need for a proactive and visionary approach. Potential for the development of mental health nursing was recognised, for example liaison mental health nursing and the opportunity for collaborative work with other members of the care-giving team. Also acknowledged was the need to promote mental health nursing as a service available to the general public and to be more visible and transparent about what it had to offer. Another issue that was recognised was the need for a review of mental health units within district general hospitals as some evidence presented to the review team suggested that such units had serious deficiencies as a therapeutic setting.

4. *Challenging issues facing mental health nurses*: There were 10 issues that were identified within this theme commencing with the belief that there was discrimination against women and that their needs were not being met. There was also a call for single sex accommodation and a choice of gender of a named nurse or key worker. The review considered that the mental health needs of children and adolescents could become problematic in later life if undetected and untreated; hence, nurses needed to be aware of family dynamics and to be able to assess situations appropriately. Also highlighted were homeless people; the needs of the elderly and their increasing numbers and under-investment in training needs of staff working with the elderly; HIV and AIDS; sexual abuse; substance misuse; the needs of mentally disordered offenders and risk assessment.

5. *Mental health nurses and research*: The review team defined the term research as a 'rigorous and systematic enquiry, conducted on a scale and using methods commensurate with the issues to be investigated, and designed to lead to more generalised contributions to knowledge' (Department of Health 1994 p37). It was recognised that not all nurses would be active in research or were equipped to be, but it was believed that all nurses should be research-aware; a vital factor if nursing is to be taken seriously as a profession with a body of research evidence that underpins its practice. However, the review acknowledged that although there was an increasing body of research produced by nurse researchers, there was still a need for strategic planning and resources for mental health nursing to really reach its potential as a generator of research. Research centres were envisaged in which research could be pursued in optimum conditions. Another innovation that was suggested was a system for the dissemination of research and other relevant information for mental health nursing that is accessible to clinical areas, possibly through the Internet. This latter point is important since many nursing libraries that were attached to hospitals have been relocated and integrated into universities.

6. *Mental health nursing: initial and continuing education*: Project 2000 (i.e. diploma and degree level pre-registration courses) aimed to provide

a knowledgeable, questioning and adaptable nurse but the review highlighted concerns relating to the balance of subjects within the Common Foundation Programme, that insufficient emphasis was being given to mental health nursing. Concern was also expressed about the duration of clinical experiences and the educational viability of brief placements. Furthermore, it was suggested that in order to maintain and to enhance the skills of the teachers of mental health nursing, they should spend at least one day a week in practice. Other concerns related to recruitment and future workforce planning, the need for appropriate post-registration education and training as well as clinical supervision that should be available to all mental health nurses. Multi-agency working was seen as a way of providing the impetus for shared learning with other health care workers. Service users were also seen as people who had a positive contribution to make both in teaching and curriculum development.

There are similarities in what the 1968 and the 1994 reviews suggest. The former emphasised the separate training and identity of the Registered Mental Nurse (RMN). The latter continued to support the notion of specialist qualification at initial pre-registration level and that mental health nursing should not become a post-registration speciality.

In summary, the 1994 review makes 42 recommendations that relate to the need for greater user and carer focus; essential focus on people with serious and enduring mental illness; the potential for mental health nursing to be at the vanguard of practice; developing advanced nursing practice (for example psychosocial intervention with people with a diagnosis of schizophrenia); developing the key worker role (now referred to as care coordinator); providing information to service users in a digestible manner; establishing systems of clinical supervision and positive leadership.

In many ways the success or failure of the review has to be looked at within its broader political context and the underlying aim of the Government to contain expenditure and rationalise services. This introduced a contradiction and undermined the political will to ensure the recommendations happened in practice. Some of the review's recommendations can be brought about by changes within education, training and practice areas at no additional cost. However, there are many issues that do require extra financial resources and there is very little discussion in the report that addressed this issue.

As a culmination of the changes occurring in the 1980s the review can be seen as the Government responding appropriately in forging ahead with the agenda for change, but parallels can be made with events from the 1960s and the 1970s and what Nolan (1993 p134) refers to as 'the era of public inquiries': 'there was a feeling amongst psychiatric nurses that the many Reports on the mental hospitals had become mere stalling tactics by governments that wanted to appear compassionate whilst spending as little money as possible on an issue that was unlikely to be a vote winner'.

IDENTIFYING MENTAL HEALTH NURSING SKILLS

The 1994 review attempted to address the problem of identifying psychiatric nurses' skills. Others have also attempted to clarify the position (Altschul (1972), Cormack (1976a 1983), Carr (1979) and Peplau (1987)) yet the issue has still not been satisfactorily addressed. The perceptual framework, in which psychiatric nursing has developed, has changed according to other dominant theories and values of the day. More precisely, psychiatric nursing has stood in the ideological shadow of psychiatric medicine, functioning mainly as a medical support system. Nonetheless, the medical model has not gone unchallenged. The psychoanalytical movement that proposed a psychological approach to mental illness was slow to make an impression on the way in which nursing was being practised, but nevertheless it did make an impression in terms of a move towards therapeutic care. The psychosocial model of Jones (1968) also began to make real inroads into how nursing was being practised with its emphasis on 'therapeutic communities'. This thinking soon gave way to behaviourism in the 1970s, that is based on the assumption that behaviour is learnt and has a purpose and that faulty learning often takes place. This was applied to psychiatric patients in attempting to help them unlearn certain behaviour and to learn more appropriate behaviour. Therefore, the necessary skills for the psychiatric nurse were those that would enable them to implement behavioural programmes. Psychodynamic and humanistic psychology with its person-centred approach and its emphasis on 'personal growth' followed in the 1980s and did win favour with many nurses who could identify with the interpersonal world of the nurse and the patient, but by and large this remained rhetoric rather than reality. In terms of the skills of the nurse, the 1982 syllabus of training identified intangibles such as self-awareness, genuineness and one's attitude as key issues. However, the broad and equivocal definition of the role of the mental health nurse from the 1968 review remained intact. A student (Duffy 1984) reflecting on the new 1982 Registered Mental Nurse (RMN) syllabus of training believed that there was an obvious need to clarify the role of the psychiatric nurse and to move away from the ideal of flexibility, 'being a jack-of-all-trades at one moment and at other occasions an efficient, empathetic and focused nurse'.

Whatever the theoretical model that is applied to nursing, it is the nurse–patient relationship that should be at the centre of nursing practice. We have seen that this has been on the psychiatric-mental health agenda for a long time, addressed by nurses and researchers as well as those that use the services. Following from the 1982 syllabus of training there was a good deal of research attempting to further clarify the proper role of the mental health nurse and suggesting reasons for the continuing failures within nursing practice. Interpersonal skills were continuously being identified as key for good mental health nursing and were intrinsic to the *Project 2000* training programmes that were introduced in the 1990s. The skills that enable nurses to engage effectively with users became identified as central for the preparation of nurses.

In 1987 the Joint Committee of Mental Health Nursing organisation had stated that 'psychiatric nursing operates within a conceptual framework of social psychiatry and that the nurse's role is characterised by a synthesis of knowledge built up from medicine, social and behavioural sciences, physiological sciences and skills training' (Barker 1990). Barker (1990 p344) cited the view of The Psychiatric Nurses Association–Scotland on the role of the psychiatric nurse and suggested that the nurse 'operates on a social model in which the emphasis is on patient–client self help; regardless of whether nurses work under a traditional medical model or social model they constitute the most important influence in the patient's social environment'. Barker (1989) back in 1989 had suggested that the first step to effectively engage with the user is to accept the pre-eminence of the person in care and suggested five rules of engagement that are still relevant today:

1. No weapons. One should not try to use one's status or position, real or imagined, to control the person in care.
2. Feel the fear. One needs to appreciate the individual's view of a problem. There is no need to explain it away.
3. Climb down from the pedestal. One needs to explore the life with its owner, to become involved, collaborate and work with the person.
4. Build a raft. A structure is required if one is not to get drowned in the sea of possibilities.
5. Help the person to embark on his/her own personal quest and be the judge and jury.

Burnard (1989) and Koshy (1989) amongst others, suggested that certain basic skills such as listening and responding supportively to people are fairly obviously helpful and need to be developed, but are, unfortunately, often commented upon for their deficiency in practice. It is important, therefore, to understand the factors that inhibit and encourage a quality nurse–user relationship and the skills that are central to quality care. Hopton (1993) suggested that 'an explanation is required about why nurses, whose motivation is generally considered as humanitarian, are manipulated into colluding with the oppression of those whose sufferings they wish to alleviate'. In endeavouring to answer this question he indicated that many users supported the thesis of psychiatry as oppression and gave examples of nurses bullying users into participating in useless social activities and of other nursing activity, which users experienced as degrading. He further suggests that the blame was not wholly with individual nurses, but that good intentions were compromised or overridden by organisational and/or ideological pressures and the contradictions that underpinned their practice.

Barker (1990 p345) suggested that British psychiatry, which in turn influences nursing, had been characterised by a broad eclectic base, and he wondered whether that eclecticism was nothing more than the desire of a child reaching out for whatever is in its grasp and quickly disregarding it in the light of the availability of another object. Counselling appeared to be a 1990s nursing 'object' and more recently psychosocial interventions with emphasis on family interventions, educational programmes for either users or carers/family members and cognitive behavioural therapy have all found favour as has training in 'control and restraint' (Sullivan 1998). The latter might suggest that psychiatric nurses are seeking refuge in its roots as custodians of the mad, bad and other marginalised individuals to whom society gives a low priority. These matters seem to reflect an identity crisis which nursing has been going through at least for the last three decades. Mental health nursing is squeezed between the orthodoxies and demands of other professional and theoretical perspectives, governments with economic agendas concerned with balancing the books and with what is immediately cost effective and the changing ideological and moral climate of the late 20th century.

THE PROFESSIONALISATION OF NURSING

The call for nursing to become a profession in its own right may be viewed as an attempt to give nursing a clearer identity and greater self-esteem. The nursing role and the skills to perform this role would be defined within a professional structure. *Project 2000* aimed to promote nursing as a profession. The nursing process was introduced as a means of giving nurses a structure and a systematic way of engaging with service users. Interpersonal and communication skills and the therapeutic use of self were promoted within this framework, which required additional skills of being able to plan and think analytically. Integral to *Project 2000*, nurses were expected to accept greater responsibility and to be prepared to develop professionally. Accountability and professionalism were concepts that had become increasingly apparent on the nursing agenda of the 1980s and 1990s, the former as defined by Hyde (1985) is, 'the ability and willingness to anticipate the results of your action and, considering those results, to act and to be held to account by your peers for those actions'. A profession, on the other hand, is a group that has specialist training and education, autonomous practice and a body of knowledge that underpins its practice (Dingwall 1974, Morrall 1998 p38). Pilgrim and Rogers (1993 p80) suggested 'the word professional tends to imply both special skills and ethical propriety. It implies competence, efficiency, altruism and integrity'. Can mental health nursing really claim to fulfil such criteria and is it able to evaluate what it does impartially and hold itself accountable for its actions?

Following the Nightingale tradition that defined the nursing role as subordinate to that of the medical doctor, the purpose of nursing was seen to be, primarily, to carry out doctor's orders. Morrall (1998 p39) cites Freidson's contention 'that since doctors control the admission of patients, they are ultimately responsible for the diagnosis and treatment, and therefore wield much influence over nursing practice'. This perception of nursing practice, as being subordinate to the doctor's professionalism, is deeply ingrained and is an enduring self-image of many nurses that negates the concept of a professional. It has been argued that the pursuit of professionalism might not be desirable. Indeed, some critical thinkers such as Goffman (1961), Illich (1977, Illich et al 1977) and Gould (1981) hold the view that too much professional control over health issues could have not only a disabling effect on users but also an iatrogenic one. Nevertheless the thrust within *Project 2000* was to endeavour to professionalise nursing. There was certainly, and still is, a case for a professional nurse with more self-esteem and autonomy and there was a strong argument that it was only from a position of credible self worth that any positive relationship or partnership with others (users) could be built. However, an increase in nurses' professional status does not guarantee any user share in the shift of power that this might entail. Hugman (1991 p1) was of the opinion that the interconnection of power and caring work in health and welfare provision had been relatively under-explored and posed the question, 'In what ways are relationships between professionals and service users, and between different professional groups, created and maintained as forms of power?' Hopton (1993) further called for an analysis of power relationships between nurses and service users if a truly user-centred partnership approach to care is to become a possibility.

Whether or not the pursuit of professionalism was considered as positive, it still remains questionable as to whether any professional status could actually become a reality for mental health nursing given its historical baggage. Five years after the introduction of *Project 2000*, Gijbels (1995) identified factors influencing the employment of skills and elicited the following from the nurses he interviewed: 'administrative duties, responding to senior management and servicing other disciplines all took priority over therapeutic (nursing) activities'. Where is the autonomous accountable practitioner in the midst of such attitudes and practice? It may be that nurses need to consider their role carefully and to avoid the tendency to either take refuge in familiar and comfortable traditional niches or to launch into an agenda for change which is concerned to present nursing as a profession in an attempt to seek power and status, losing sight of the real difference that nursing can make to improve the quality of mental health services, through a proper identification of how nurses in practice can develop partnership working and fulfil a meaningful, qualitative and effective role.

Education as an agent of change

Project 2000 had been acclaimed as an opportunity for nursing to put its house in order with greater emphasis on higher education in line with other professionals and the pursuit of diploma and degree level qualifications. One of the questions that Onega (1991) posed in her study of a theoretical framework for psychiatric nursing practice was; what is the primary factor that influences each psychiatric nurse's style of nursing practice? The answer she gave was that it depended on the individual's ability to think logically, abstractly, concretely and clearly about nursing phenomena. Stevenson (1988), in regard to education and knowledge, suggests that 'knowledge changes one's thinking process. One's thinking process influences behaviour. Therefore, nursing knowledge changes nursing practice'. Thus great store was placed on education as an agent for changing nursing culture. However, the optimism was not unanimous. Orr (1990) who in 1990 examined published work over a 20-year period, suggested that, 'the nursing profession today is as traditional as it was in the 1960s'. Daniels (1990) also referred to many of the problems in nursing as being associated with inflexibility and the defence of the status quo rather than with concerns about changes within mental health services within the context of user needs and the quality of care. With the conservatism in nursing that is resistant to change, how could the conflict between practices, emanating from traditional roots and the education and training of nurses, with students more receptive to new ideas, be resolved? This is often referred to as the 'theory/practice gap' and can give rise to role conflict, the development of negative attitudes, loss of job satisfaction and problems in recruiting and retaining nurses.

The National Foundation for Educational Research (NFER) (1990 pp3–4) that surveyed the first 6 ENB pilot schemes of *Project 2000* reported that:

- There is a need to remain aware of the time scales involved in introducing change.
- There is a need to establish and maintain effective communications, an open management ethos and a shared commitment to innovation across all sectors and at all levels.
- There is a need to be alert and sensitive to the psychosocial aspects of change and inter-organisational collaboration.

Then again, how long do service users have to wait for changes to become more user focused? The issue of integrating taught theory into practice and the anxieties of students about to take on 'registered nurse' responsibilities were also reported as examples of concerns in the study. Hence, there was some concern with the speed of change, which if allowed to go unregulated 'may actually increase role conflict by forcing traditionalists into a defensive authoritarian stance when faced with new research and the problem solving orientated student nurse' (Orr 1990 p60).

The growth of an intellectual tradition in nursing has been slow but the changing baseline qualification at diploma level for nurses and the pursuit of degree level qualifications may help this process along and produce a nursing workforce that is more responsive to the needs of users. The introduction of the Post-Registration Education and Practice Programme (PREPP) by the UKCC (United Kingdom Central Council for Nursing, Midwifery and Health Visiting 1997) also appeared to be a step in the right direction in endeavouring to ensure that practitioners do not remain within a culture of relative static knowledge and that they must keep up to date in order to be safe practitioners. Emphasis has also been given to the need for advanced nursing practice to support and build up nursing professional status. The UKCC stated that advanced practice is concerned with:

- Adjusting the boundaries for the development of future practice.
- Pioneering and developing new roles that are responsive to changing needs.
- Advancing clinical practice, research and education to enrich nursing practice as a whole.
- Contributing to health policy and management and the

determination of health needs.

- Continuing the development of the professional in the interests of patients, clients and health service.

From this position it was envisaged that there would be innovations and research-based practice, experts who have a consultancy role, high level professional leadership and increased political influence plus expert resources within education, supervision and management. Such individuals were likely to be educated to either Masters or Doctoral level. Clinton and Nelson (1999) have suggested that the term 'advanced practice' is often taken to refer to technical skills that are difficult to acquire, and moreover, to require knowledge that would normally be gained in studying for a higher degree'. However, they further define advanced nursing practice as, 'second order reflection that brings into question the assumptions on which such technical interventions are based. If day to day practice is a first order activity in which the everyday understandings of the practitioner link theory and practice in the immediate sense of the judgements and beliefs embedded in practice, second order reflection is the process of scrutinising and challenging these conceptualisations'. Therefore, advanced practice is taken to mean the reflective skills involved in examining ways of thinking about mental health interventions.

Towards the closing years of the 20th century there was much criticism being directed at nurse preparation and in 1999 the Commission for Education made it clear that the current curriculum model of four branches of nursing needed reviewing. In the same year the government launched *Making a Difference – Strengthening the nursing, midwifery and health visiting contribution to health and health care* (Department of Health 1999b) and suggested that there is a need to increase the level of nurses practical skills, to ensure that education is more responsive to the National Health Service, a need to promote leadership and to devise programmes that enable nurses to be flexible and adapt to change. The ENB also called for programmes to be restructured so that the common foundation programme is only of one-year duration and the branch of two years with 50% of the programme practice based. It was also suggested that the level of award on completion of nurse education courses in all four countries needs to reflect the complexity of nursing and equivalence with other professions and graduate preparation at the point of registration should be expanded to all of the four countries of the UK. The extent to which the current changes taking place within nurse preparation and the health care system can cause lasting and effective positive change remains to be seen and it might be argued that education can enhance confidence that may be used by vested interests to defend the status quo rather than change it.

SUMMARY

In considering the major government reviews of mental health nursing that have been conducted during the last 30 years, it is interesting to note that there is much in common between the 1968 and the 1994 reviews, but unfortunately real change has been slow in coming. The 1968 review saw the role of the nurse as diverse but mainly about keeping the users occupied, although it also mentioned the need for nursing to become more therapeutic in its endeavour, to engage in research and to identify good practices. The skills and attitudes desirable for a mental health nurse were fundamentally to treat those in their care as individuals, to have effective listening skills, clear communication and to tend to physical and personal hygiene. Furthermore, the role of the nurse was regarded as synthesised from psychodynamic, behavioural, social, physiological and medical perspectives. It is not surprising that some of the interim literature suggested that mental health nursing was a 'Jack of all trades' that needed to discover its identity. The 1968 review implicitly suggests an attempt to compromise with the nurse's traditional role. It did not challenge sufficiently past premises or acknowledge the fundamental contradictions inherent in the different perspectives, and thus was not a solid enough basis for practical change.

The 1994 review emphasised many of the above issues but went further in promoting the need for therapeutic relationships and the role of the nurse in the context of accountability. Stemming from this, the review highlighted the issue of staffing levels. Two key issues were identified: firstly, the need to employ support staff to relieve nurses of non-nursing duties (although this had also been recommended in the 1968 review) and secondly, overall staffing levels and the need for continuity of staff to develop genuine therapeutic relationships. Other issues given greater emphasis in the 1994 review were the need to make information more freely available so that users can make real choices and the need for a greater focus on the individual, especially those with a 'serious or enduring mental illness'. However, this latter point has become an issue of contention, with Barker and Jackson (1997) suggesting that many mental health problems might be defined as severe or serious and that the 'severe and serious' adjectives have become synonymous with the diagnosis of schizophrenia. Therefore, they argue, there is a danger that mental health nurses are being encouraged to blur their boundaries and this could lead to the demise of mental health nursing.

The 1994 review also considered nursing as an autonomous profession and to this end looks at 'advanced nursing practice' in relation to psychosocial interventions. However, the report does not indicate what exactly this is and there has been a lot of debate in attempting to define 'advanced nursing practice' and whether or not nursing can really be regarded as an autonomous profession. It is evident that the pace of change within the practice of nursing is slow due to its conservatism and traditionalism as a support system for medicine. Power relationships within service provision need to change if nurses are to become authentic, accountable, autonomous practitioners; few examples exist where nurses have been able to effectively challenge the system. Whether a more educative approach to the preparation of nurses and the notion of life-long learning will help in breaking the mould remains to be seen.

The nursing agenda laid down by the 1994 review succumbed to political pressure and one can see a certain degree of a reversal in emphasis away from therapeutic interventions and community care back to institutions (hospitals with locked wards and the growth of Regional Secure Units) and concerns with social control. One must not forget the political and ideological context in which mental health services are provided and the social control arguments that writers such as Laing (1968), Szasz (1971), Lader (1977) and Scull (1979) amongst others have identified. The Draft Mental Health Bill (Department of Health 2002) also raised a lot of concern: if the new laws were to be passed, many innocent people could be at risk of being detained indefinitely just because they have mental health problems and are deemed to be at risk of committing a crime. With the focus upon dangerousness and risk, the danger to users is that it can add to the stigma and prejudice they experience, compounding difficulties in securing housing and employment. Others could be forced to take medication, even if the side-effects are too horrendous to bear; there is currently much emphasis being given to compliance with medication that could mean a removal of choice and deter people from seeking mental health services support. The provisions for user involvement are also minimal and people may feel unable to exercise their right to refuse unwanted medical treatment if they have been forcibly taken to a place for the purpose of receiving that treatment. An over-reliance on medication that can have serious and long-lasting side effects could prevail and it could operate unfairly against black and ethnic minority groups as they are more likely to be diagnosed mentally ill and are more likely to be compulsorily detained under the Mental Health Act (Rogers & Pilgrim 1996 p138). There are also concerns regarding breaching human rights and for the person to be released from this power, one must prove that supervision is no longer required rather than the doctor having to prove that it continues to be. Fortunately it appears that the government is rethinking some of its proposals within the Draft Mental Health Bill, as the subject was not mentioned in the Queen's speech as a topic for the agenda for the 2003 Parliamentary session.

Although the present Government has made a commitment to quality outcomes that involve the voice of the service user, other political pressures are evident, such as the perceived populist appeal to safeguard society from dangerous individuals. There appears to be a see-sawing from care of patients to protection of the public and risk reduction through containment through physical or chemical means. This is a real dilemma for society: do we care for disturbed and distressed individuals or should we lock them up? This in turn has implications for how we educate and train those who we put in their charge. The Mental Health Task Force was set up to spearhead an improved mental health service that is responsive to the needs of users, but whether the rhetoric of empowerment and consumerism and what that implies becomes reality in practice, remains to be seen.

Elston (1991) suggests that the past decade has witnessed the end of the era of the passive patient, but the very notion of moving from a professionally (psychiatrist) led service to one that is based on power sharing can be challenging and, for some, inordinately threatening. Control to a certain extent has been decentralised and we have witnessed over the past decade the rise of the individual, the promotion of empowerment and partnership in care and an attack on professional control. Nurses can no longer remain subservient or servants of routine; they are now being expected to be accountable practitioners and to engage with the whole person, their strengths and deficits. The process of empowering users can also consolidate the nursing position and role. However, there is a danger that the nursing agenda can be one in which the pursuit of professional status transcends the needs of users of mental health services.

This chapter aims to provide a solid base on which to further explore the role of mental health nursing in the context of meeting the perceived needs of users of mental health services, the extent to which some of the identified issues are now obsolete, to refocus on significant issues and to consider areas that have not been addressed. A more detailed and contemporary understanding of both users' and nursing perceptions is required, given the proposed and real changes within mental health services. A study of this nature is important at a time when collaboration and partnership issues are high on the health care agenda, with a need to ensure that resources are used to maximum effect in providing a modern and dependable service that has the user at the centre of its endeavour.

References

Altschul A 1972 Patient-nurse interactions: a study of interaction patterns in acute psychiatric wards. Churchill Livingstone, Edinburgh

Barker P 1989 Rules of engagement. Nursing Times 85(51):58-60

Barker P 1990 The conceptual basis of mental health nursing. Nurse Education Today 10:339-348

Barker P, Jackson S 1997 Mental health nursing: making it a primary concern. Nursing Standard 11(17):39-41

Burnard P 1989 Fads and fashions. Nursing Times 85(2):70

Carr P 1979 To describe the role of the psychiatric nurse in a psychiatric unit, which is situated in a district general hospital complex. PhD thesis. University of Manchester, Manchester

Clinton M, Nelson S 1999 Advanced practice in mental health nursing. Blackwell Science, Oxford

Cormack D 1976 Psychiatric nursing observed. Royal College of Nursing, London

Cormack D 1983 Psychiatric nursing described. Churchill Livingstone, Edinburgh

Daniels G 1990 Ten steps to better practice. Nursing Times 86(11):72

Department of Health 1994 Working in partnership. Report of the Mental Health Nursing Review Team. HMSO, London

Department of Health 1999a Press release: Committee of Inquiry into the Personality Disorder Unit, Ashworth Special Hospital, no.2. HMSO, London

Department of Health 1999b Making a difference: strengthening the nursing, midwifery and health visiting contribution to health and health care. Department of Health, London

Department of Health 2002 The draft Mental Health Bill. Department of Health, London

Dingwall R 1974 Some sociological aspects of nursing research. Sociological Review 22(1):44-45

Duffy D 1984 A student's view. Nursing Times 80(30):67-68

Elston M A 1991 The politics of professional power: medicine in a changing health service. In: Gabe J, Calnan M, Bury M (eds) The sociology of the health service, ch 3. Routledge, London

Ferguson K, Brooker C 1996 Mental health nursing: a review of the literature. School of Nursing, University of Manchester

Gijbels H 1995 Mental health nursing skills in an acute admission environment: perceptions of mental health nurses and other mental health professionals. Journal of Advanced Nursing 21:460-465

Goffman E 1961 Asylums. Penguin, Harmondsworth

Gould A 1981 The salaried middle class in the corporate welfare state. Policy and Politics 9(4):401-408

Hopton J 1993 The contradictions of mental health nursing. Nursing Standard 8(11):37-39

Hugman R 1991 Power in the caring professions. Macmillan,

Basingstoke

Hyde P 1985 Accountability. Nursing Mirror 160(16):24

Illich I 1977 Limits to medicine. Penguin, Harmondsworth

Illich I, Zola I K, McKnight J (eds) 1977 Disabling professions. Marion Boyars, London

Jones M 1968 Psychiatry in practice: the ideas of the therapeutic community. Penguin, Harmondsworth

Koshy K T 1989 I only have ears for you. Nursing Times 85(30):26

Lader M 1977 Psychiatry on trial. Penguin, Harmondsworth

Laing R D 1967 The politics of experience. Penguin, Harmondsworth

McMillan I 1997 Special assignment. Mental Health Practice 1(1):8-9

Martin J P 1984 Hospitals in trouble. Blackwell, London

Ministry of Health 1962 A hospital plan for England and Wales. Cmnd 1604. HMSO, London

Ministry of Health/Central Health Services Council 1968 Psychiatric nursing today and tomorrow. Report of the Joint Sub-committee of the Standing Mental Health and Standing Nursing Advisory Committees. HMSO, London

Morrall P 1998 Mental health nursing and social control. Whurr, London

Murphy E 1991 After the asylums. Faber and Faber, London

National Foundation for Educational Research 1990 Charting the course: a study of the 6 ENB pilot schemes in preregistration nurse education. National Foundation for Educational Research 3-4

Nolan P 1993 A history of mental health nursing. Chapman and Hall, London

Onega L L 1991 A theoretical framework for psychiatric nursing practice. Journal of Advanced Nursing 16:68-73

Orr J G 1990 Tradition v Project 2000 - something old something new. Nurse Education Today 10:58-62

Peplau H 1987 Tomorrow's world. Nursing Times 83(1):29-32

Pilgrim D, Rogers A 1993 A sociology of mental health and illness. OUP, Buckingham

Rogers A, Pilgrim D 1996 Mental health policy in Britain: a critical introduction. Macmillan, Basingstoke

Rogers A, Pilgrim D, Lacey R 1993 Experiencing psychiatry: users' views of services. Macmillan/MIND, London

Scull A 1979 Museums of madness. RKP, London

Stevenson J S 1988 Nursing knowledge development: into era II. Journal of Professional Nursing 4(3):152-162

Sullivan P 1998 Care and control in mental health nursing. Nursing Standard 13(15):42-45

Szasz T 1971 The manufacturing of madness. RKP, London

United Kingdom Central Council for Nursing, Midwifery and Health Visiting 1997 PREP and you. UKCC, London

Zito J, Howlett M 1996 Introduction. In: Sheppard D (ed) Learning the lessons, 2nd edn. The Zito Trust, London

Chapter 3

User perspectives

INTRODUCTION

This chapter begins with an exploration of the rise and development of a user movement and user perspectives. It considers the views expressed by users and ex-users during the 1980s concerning their experiences of treatment and how they identify their own needs. It looks at the users' criticism of the current situation within mental health services and how it is challenging the way people work. It is important to establish why a user movement developed and to consider why partnership is now on the ascendancy. There appears to be very little published on user issues prior to the 1980s but since then many users have been writing about their own experiences.

In 1988 a report that involved 100 service users, published jointly by Camden Mental Health Consortium (CMHC) and Good Practice in Mental Health (GPMH) service user groups, entitled *Treated Well? A Code of Practice for Psychiatric Hospitals* concluded that many people find a stay in hospital to be unhelpful and or even damaging. The report was mainly concerned with attitudes rather than resources. Some of the findings showed that, particularly for women, 'psychiatric hospital wards were not very safe places and that the initial hospital stay was generally found to be upsetting and often devaluing' (Camden Mental Health Consortium 1988 p5). Regrettably this is still an issue of concern and the following are other issues raised by users in the CMHC study:

- There was a complete lack of information. I was bundled about from one place to another with no information about what was happening.
- I felt helpless and forced into a system that lost my identity.
- A nurse filled in a form, she was very efficient and in a hurry. I felt a nuisance.
- The nurses were always too busy.
- Staff appeared to avoid normal ways of behaving. When they meet you in the corridor, even if they know you, they seldom acknowledge you. They do not even acknowledge distress, if you were upset the last time they met you they never ask you how you are (Camden Mental Health Consortium 1988 p13).

The latter comments have echoes of Menzies study, *Social Systems as a Defence Against Anxiety* where she describes the nurse–patient relationship and suggests that, '... the core of the anxiety situation for the nurse lies in the relationship with the patient. The closer and more concentrated the relationship, the more the nurse is likely to experience the impact of anxiety' (Menzies-Lyth 1970 p11). The best way of avoiding such anxiety is therefore not to get too involved with service users and to be occupied doing other more mundane tasks. Fielding and Llewelyn (1986) also shared the view that many nurses failed to develop interpersonal skills and genuine therapeutic relationships because they actively avoided close relationships as an attempt to defend themselves from emotional distress. Restricted contact can be an effective defence mechanism for resolving possible emotionally charged situations.

The following comments from the 1988 report also serve to indicate the unequal relationship that users of the services experience:

- Ward rounds are so indelicate in the way they are conducted, because they are only for the benefit of the staff and consultants. They are like an interrogation, trial by multi-disciplinary team.
- My rights were not explained to me.
- The damage done by ward rounds is far more harmful than the benefits. Most of the staff there do not speak. Anyway, what do people know when they have not met you before, except perhaps for a few minutes? (Camden Mental Health Consortium 1988 p17)

More specific criticisms were that qualified staff spent too much time in the office, where users were not welcomed. Too many agency staff were used, the least experienced and students particularly were left with responsibility for interacting with users. Furthermore, it was reported that many professionals did not have sufficient skills in listening, counselling and problem solving. The report saw nurses as being the key people in mental health services as they are the ones who have the greatest amount of contact with service users. Accordingly, mental health nurses could be of the greatest support but the majority of users did not feel that their needs were being met or taken seriously. Although what one might be hearing in these accounts is the result of an unreflective and unresponsive system, staff may have said similar things about how users were treated. If mental health workers have not been educated or supervised to cope with failure in themselves or others, then the system that prepares them and within which they work, has to take some of the responsibility for failing users.

Nevertheless, in response to the findings, CMHC and GPMH set out to influence the quality of the services by compiling a Code of Practice for Psychiatric Hospitals, within the report, with 70 recommendations for responding to the needs of service users. The essence of the recommendations was that users should be allowed to negotiate their own care and treatment and, where necessary, challenge professionals. The conclusion of the report emphasised and put forward the questions, why should a stay in hospital be such an unhelpful experience? and, why do professionals find it so difficult to empathise with the people placed in their care?

To begin to answer these questions one must consider the historic definition of mental illness and how, in the past, society has dealt with the problem. Historically, individuals who exhibited irrational and disturbing behaviour outside of the accepted norms of society were incarcerated for the benefit of that society, not for the individual with the problems. Once incarcerated, the individuals could be acted upon or treated. Systems evolved around this definition and with these political agendas, vested interests and power bases. These systems also helped to define the attitudes of the individuals who worked within them. Ideological shifts in western thought have given rise to new concerns about 'mental illness' which are centred around the individual's subjective feelings of well being and thus the focus is on effective communication, therapeutic relationships and partnership working. This shift in perspective involves undermining the past orthodoxy.

A report by the Islington Mental Health Forum (IMHF) in 1989 also describes how, in one particular hospital, users found that treatment was exclusively with psychotropic medication. The issues that concerned these users were related to choice, individuality and the lack of different treatment modalities. These concerns can be made much more real and vivid by looking at some of the verbatim responses. On the question of choice: 'it is nil for mental health service users'; individuality: 'there is a tendency to see people as cases'; symptoms: 'we are not considered to have individual needs'; treatment input: 'only tokenism, a real input into planning is required' (Islington Mental Health Forum 1989 p9).

These responses were critical of the system. Users had a view and could provide it if they were consulted. They saw themselves as having a wealth of experience and a body of knowledge gained through using mental health services. However, to have any real choice they also needed information about treatment interventions and felt that treatment should not equate simply with medication. They expressed concern that they were being seen as 'psychiatric patients' first rather than as 'people' with mental health problems and this, they suggested, affected the way in which service providers responded to them. That response was often perceived by users as being negative: 'I am a human being first. Being a patient is just a part of my life and sometimes there is an increase in passivity quite simply due to the lack of any point in talking or arguing if no one listens, or takes any notice of what you are saying' (Islington Mental Health Forum 1989 p22). As a result of these criticisms the IMHF suggested that planning must be based on users' actual needs and no longer on what professionals and society believe their needs to be. They considered that working in partnership should prevail, whereby users' views and feelings are taken into account when any treatment intervention, decisions and care plan were being devised.

Many of the issues being identified by service users fitted into themes that suggested a power struggle and the need to challenge the way in which the mental health systems were organised. Rogers and Pilgrim (1991) identified the following themes:

- Reversing marginalisation and powerlessness
- Challenging the consensus set by others and
- Challenging authoritative views on mental health.

The following comments by one user are a poignant expression of the dichotomy existing between the treatment experienced for mental health problems and the sort of help users actually want from the service:

> 'As a survivor of the psychiatric services, in the name of care and medicine I have been locked up, drugged and subjected to ceremonial degradation. Some of the treatments I received caused greater problems than those identified as my symptoms when I started my psychiatric career'. (Pembroke 1991)

The value system this user encountered was one of oppression, whereby she was expected to be a good and grateful patient, conducting herself without expressing her anger, being submissive, subservient and dressing neatly and tidily. Insight meant agreeing with the professionals. Her distress was only acknowledged in the context of a medical model of psychiatry and her worldview and experiences of living were largely unimportant. She felt that her distress was being medicalised for the benefit of the pharmacological industry. The treatment offered seemed to be that she had to fit into what was there, on the provider's terms, rather than the provider attempting to make sense of her distress and responding accordingly. Her experience reflected concerns similar to those expressed by Illich (1977) who suggested that 'the medical establishment has become a major threat to health. The disabling impact of professional control over medicine has reached the proportions of an epidemic'. A decade later Shields et al (1988) also concluded that 'Patients are passive recipients of a service provided by professionals and deficiencies will continue until the patients are allowed to take more control of their lives whilst in the health care delivery system'. McIntyre et al (1989) reported similar findings and showed that what patients valued most about being in hospital was their ability to leave. Drug treatment was seen to be only 'quite' helpful and more attention was desired for problem solving approaches and talking therapies.

The move to community care was potentially a means to greater user empowerment. Small-scale residential homes and day centres away from hospital sites were being asked for by users, plus care in their own homes. However, Lindow (1993) suggested that 'one barrier to progress is the fear of some professional people that change means they will lose their roles. This sometimes results in services still being provided in institutionalised ways in the community'. Nevertheless, Holloway (1988) looked at day care services and showed that 65% of the users were appreciative and positive about the service in that it gave them the opportunity to meet people and to socialise, thereby alleviating loneliness whilst the activities kept the mind occupied. There was little mention of any systematic behavioural or psychotherapeutic interventions. It appeared that most of these people were on the margins of society, they were lonely, unemployed and used the service in a way that others in employment use their work to meet people and therefore were much more integrated into communities and society at large.

Hogman and Melzer (1992) in their study consulted 140 users diagnosed as suffering from schizophrenia about their opinion of the care they received, and the issues that they identified of greatest concern were similar to the findings of Holloway (1988). Accommodation, money and the need for employment and/or occupation were their priorities. There was confusion over professional roles, such as mistaking a Community Psychiatric Nurse (CPN) for a Social Worker, and the input expected tended to be advice on housing, welfare benefits, retraining courses and jobs. Their role as a friend or companion was also more often sought. The overall findings from Hogman and Melzer (1992) indicate that when people with a mental health problem were asked how they would improve their care they referred to basic needs associated with everyday living that all of us should be able to recognise. Users did not specifically focus on their illness identity or diagnosis as being of paramount concern. Very often service users perceived mental health care to be focused on control of their psychiatric symptoms and of the risk associated with behavioural disturbance, rather than on what they themselves viewed as more fundamental quality-of-life issues.

Barker and Walters (1993) looked at an urban community-based psychiatric service and compared the views of the users with those of the community nurses providing them, and suggested that users perceived less choice and options, information and involvement in their care and treatment than the nurse subjects. Despite this, they suggested that users were generally less critical of the available services than the nurses, although this may have indicated that user responses could be affected by their position as disempowered service users currently in the system, dependent on services and fearing comeback and rejection. The study identified what intervention users found most useful from nurses. However, the project did make a distinction between measuring the therapeutic efficacy of the Clinical Nurse Specialist (CNS) and the generic Community Psychiatric Nurse (CPN). The former had undergone training in behavioural psychotherapy and was perceived as a more therapeutic agency with a strong emphasis upon 'confronting reality' and practising 'behaviour change'. The generic CPNs were appreciated more for basic 'human qualities' and scored higher on issues such as showing understanding, helping with medication, giving direct answers and clients feeling that the nurses 'just liked them' (Barker & Walters 1993 pp6–7). The interventions users found most useful were as follows:

CNSs
- Helping the patient to face up to reality.
- Explaining the relationship of the patient's present problems to earlier life events.
- Helping the patient see others as possessing similar problems.
- Helping the patient to understand him or herself.
- Encouraging the patient to practise certain behaviours.
- Encouraging homework assignments.
- Assisting the patient to set goals.
- Teaching the patient relaxation techniques.
- Promoting life changes.
- Expecting more mature behaviour of the patient.
- Discussing the patient's feelings.

CPNs
- Patient felt s/he was talking to an understanding person.
- The patient felt that his/her confidence was restored.
- The nurse helped the patient with medication.
- The patient felt that the nurse 'just liked me'.
- The nurse always gave direct answers.

The study did not compare the different type of interventions of the two groups in terms of which users valued most. From the above identified interventions, one can appreciate the notion of a helping relationship and that users did focus upon the quality of relationships, particularly in the case of the CPNs. Holyoake (1997) amongst others has reported that 'such is the importance of helping relationships that mental health nursing has at the heart of its practice the use of the therapeutic self'. If nurse contact and relationship building is central to this practice then much importance must be placed upon nurses and users having the opportunity to actually spend time together. Sadly many comments within current literature still suggest that health care professionals do not spend sufficient time engaging with users.

If users consider human relationships as central to their definition of a quality service it is not surprising that inadequate communication has been an issue that is constantly on users' agendas in particular, as it relates to giving information, but change in response to this has been very slow in coming (Brandon 1991, Essex et al 1990, Health Service Commissioner for England, Scotland and Wales 1993). Brandon (1991) tells us that he was admonished by a consultant psychiatrist for giving a patient the information that she had requested about the medication she was taking. This could reflect professionals' own insecurity as to their knowledge base, an issue that professionals still need to examine. Communication between users and professionals appears to be underpinned by a culture of control and defensiveness. Often professionals use language that implies that they 'own' patients, for example the use of such terms as 'my patients' and the corollary that tends to follow, 'do not worry, I am in control, you do what I suggest'.

Users' experiences on information giving suggest that they feel that professionals attempt to have a monopoly on knowledge and that they think they know best what information they should impart (Rogers et al 1993).

Part of the problem is that the public agenda for user involvement does not necessarily match that of those who work in the services, whose resistance to the public agenda for change may emanate from their own overt and covert agendas. One must remain aware of the wider issues of power, history and politics. One of the possible consequences of user involvement is that there will be winners and losers in terms of shifting power and other relationships. Hence a clear agenda for change is required that includes a strategy for influencing changes in attitudes and behaviour of the staff providing the services. The continuing changes taking place within education and training plus the fact that community care is still high on the political agenda may influence the necessary shift in attitudes. Such a shift may also be influenced by user views. Recommendation 32 of the Report of the Mental Health Nursing Review (Department of Health 1994), published in 1994, hoped to contribute to user empowerment by promoting the conviction that the people who use services and their carers should participate in teaching and in curriculum development. Although such involvement is being encouraged, we still have to ask ourselves, to what extent is this really happening today?

The closure of the large institutions and the decline in the 'jobs for life' culture has meant that psychiatric nursing has also been deconstructed and, as yet, has not been reconstructed given the fundamental changes that are currently underway within mental health services. There are many negative views being expressed by users within the literature but one has to be careful not to be left with the conclusion that mental health staff are power-crazed, sadistic and waging terror at every opportunity. Leary and Brown's (1995) findings from the Claybury study into ward-based psychiatric nursing suggested that 'nurses experience high levels of emotional exhaustion due to the demands of their work. They appeared to experience greater feelings of depersonalisation or detachment from users and less of a sense of personal accomplishment with their work compared to their community based counterparts'. Although many of the large Victorian hospitals have since closed, it does not follow that the culture and attitudes that developed in these settings have changed as a result of closure. The question is, why do some organisations perpetuate such cultures and seem unable to do much about it?

USER GROUPS – PRESSURE FOR CHANGE

The dissatisfaction has been the focus for the establishment of user groups, through which a meaningful challenge to the traditional structures of mental health could be mounted. The arrival on the scene of user groups, which appear to be a phenomenon of the last 15–20 years, although the roots of their action go back much further, is challenging the traditional power base of psychiatry. Users are no longer prepared to be passive patients. A British mental health users movement can be traced back to the 1980s (Lindow 1990, Rogers & Pilgrim 1993) although the embryonic user movement was regarded as being anti-psychiatry and unrepresentative of ordinary service users. They continue to gather momentum, via groups such as the United Kingdom Advocacy Network, MIND, Survivors Speak Out, Hearing Voices Network, Mad Pride, ECT Anonymous, the National Black Mental Health Association and US – The All Wales User Network, amongst others. These are organisations that set out to improve contact and communication between user groups and individuals who are working to increase the involvement of users in the shaping of the psychiatric system. However, the user movement required a favourable climate in which to be effective and reasons for this growth in user groups included the rise of the political right in the 1980s with its dislike of welfare state dependency and approval of consumerism. Other reasons for the growth in user groups were the role of the market, the emergence of philosophies that emphasise involvement, the struggle for equal opportunities, successful action by groups in other countries, the break up of the large institutions and some success from user activity. However, to a certain extent the notion of a user movement could be regarded as a misnomer since there is not one voice that represents their position but many. Pluralism can be regarded as a normal and healthy aspect of any human struggle for change, but Campbell (1996) identifies a difficulty with this plurality of user groups in considering what criteria should be used for involvement and which user groups service providers should involve and listen to. Furthermore, many service providers feel that user organisations are unrepresentative, that they voice the wishes of the most articulate, the radical and the least ill.

Nevertheless, one cannot ignore the fact that user groups have become more organised, articulate, informed and challenging to the psychiatric system that has traditionally set itself up as 'knowing best'. They are challenging the idea that there is superior professional knowledge that should not be questioned and that the professionals know best about users' needs. Despite some of the differences of opinions between user groups, it is the issue of dignity and having a voice that can be heard that connects the different factions. The Sainsbury Centre for Mental Health (SCMH) (2003) suggest that the user movement is still expanding rapidly; more than half have a paid worker and democratic structures. Many have representation on service planning bodies and provide some form of advocacy, mutual support, education and training.

User groups are also very keen to develop opportunities for partnership to influence policy formation, planning and hence appropriate services that reflect their perceived needs based upon their experiences of the current services. There may be more and more tension between users and the providers of services, but having allies within the service is an important variable in terms of the degree of influence exercised by marginalised groups. Offe (1984) has suggested that the success and demarcation of new social movements from old social movements of the 19th century are that they are not derived solely from marginalised social groups. Instead they include members from more powerful groups who also play a central role in the management and functioning of welfare. Stilwell (1990) in addressing this issue states that 'The most lasting and revolutionary changes paradoxically do not come from revolution at all, but through the gradual evolution of ideas and attitudes until a new level of awareness demands change'.

As groups expand and different factions emerge, conflict is inevitable. The debate within the American psychiatric survivors movement has been about separatism. This involves an argument about how to retain one's own integrity and to avoid having the group's principles and aims diluted by collaboration with the established power base and their vested interests. The question of whether user groups should attempt to influence existing services, and participate in them, or work independently to establish alternatives, is a key concern. Similarly in Britain pluralism prevails and there are fundamentally different camps with respect to that question. Users want to plan and manage their own services and in the 1990s more and more proposals for self-help alternatives to mental health services were being promoted. It is possible that if the existing services fail to change sufficiently, different service providers will enter the market to provide a service that is far more user friendly and orientated. The Health Committee Report (1994), *Better Off In The Community?* put forward the view that 'there is some support for the development of user-run and managed services, including self-help groups and support networks'. It was suggested that user-led services were more flexible, responsive, less bureaucratic, appropriate and focused more on the needs of the individual within a context of their everyday lives. However, some view such developments with cynicism. A question that was posed at a user-organised conference in Wales was, 'Is this empowerment or exploitation?' since users involved in working and running certain services are usually either volunteers or self-helpers in receipt of supplementary benefits. Dodd (1998) suggests that 'there may be a novelty aspect to empowerment, which allows creative ideas to be acceptable, but on a more worrying note it may be a way of reducing dependence upon an already under-resourced and over-used service'. However, despite this cynicism, the fact remains that users are at least working and running services that they have developed to satisfy their needs from their perspective.

Users clearly do want different services and have been concerned that under the current 1983 Mental Health Act people can be compelled to use services that users may feel are not in their best interest. Lindow (1993 p3) maintains that despite some user participation in the planning of services, 'what is proving difficult is to get action on what users say, even when extensive consultation takes place'. If services are to change and become more user orientated then when users feed back to service providers, their views must not only be listened to, but also acted upon and the balance of power must shift towards a genuine collaborative approach to care. In 1983 the Griffiths Report (1983) had commented about the difficulties in hearing the authentic voice of the ultimate consumer of psychiatric services and suggested that health care should be measured by how it is perceived by users. The notion of collaboration and partnership has been firmly placed on the agenda for change and is a clear challenge to professionals who traditionally have dictated what is to happen to users.

The question that arises from the challenge posed to existing mental health services by user groups is, do the professionals have the courage and/or the political will to act on the information that is available, not just as individuals but in a corporate manner if the views of service users and proposed changes are to be taken seriously? Questions that Shields (1985) posed over almost two decades ago are still relevant and still need to be grappled with: 'We must ask ourselves how much we actually do know about users' views of the services we provide. We must also ask whether we want to know, and whether we can be flexible enough to admit that the user may know better than the professional what is best for them'. Foucault (1967) had raised this same concern over three and a half decades ago. He had much to say about society's unwillingness to engage people with mental illnesses. For him it was much more than finding out what people wanted, it was about ensuring that the system delivered in meeting real needs for housing, occupations, regular income and the opportunity to become socially and psychologically settled as a result of having such needs met. Only then can we claim that people with mental health problems have been integrated into the community/society.

Nevertheless, over the last two decades there has been a greater focus upon the views of those that use mental health services. The Mental Health Task Force, which was set up in 1993 by the Department of Health to spearhead improvements in the quality of mental health services, had on its agenda the need to listen to service users, to ensure that services are designed to meet users' and carers' needs and to ensure that providers of services deliver what they say they are going to deliver. Policy makers have accepted that user views matter and it is important that we understand why this is so. Shields (1985) suggested that there are three main reasons why users' views on their care and treatment should be sought, and these reasons are still valid today:

- A moral reason: Users are usually a vulnerable group, often frightened, unassertive and inarticulate.
- Technical and economic factors: In order to provide the most effective interventions and treatments their views provide one measure of their usefulness hence such views could lead to an improvement in the service and give better value for money.
- Political aspect: In a democracy it is the right of citizens that publicly supported services be accountable to them. Participation is a way to achieve accountability and would help to reduce the feelings of alienation that service users often experience and negate the 'us and them' resentment that is often present.

The Audit Commission's annual report regularly puts forward the view that listening to users is important if professionals and service managers are to avoid falling into the trap of making assumptions on other people's behalf, since their views often differ widely from those of service users. It has also been suggested by the National Health Service Executive (1996) that appropriate and effective services were more likely to be developed if they were planned on the basis of needs identified in conjunction with users. They suggested that there was some evidence that involving users in their own care improved health care outcomes and increased user satisfaction. This confirmed the earlier findings of Miller and Rose (1986) who suggested that devising therapeutic schemes in which clients had a share in their own care had better outcomes than those that had not.

One of the aims set out in the World Health Organization (WHO) (1986) document *Targets for Health for All* stated as one of its goals, 'the attainment by all citizens of the world by the year 2000 of a level of health that will permit them to lead a socially and economically productive life and Primary Health Care, with participation by the people is the key to this goal'. This may have been a rather idealistic goal but nevertheless a goal worthy of pursuit. Launching the consultation paper on quality at the NHS Confederation Conference in July 1998 the Secretary of State for Health announced that:

'The Government is putting quality at the heart of the new NHS We are doing something that no Government has ever done. New mechanisms to set standards, deliver standards and monitor standards. The Government is not prepared to leave quality in the NHS to chance. We will carry out an annual independent survey of the experience of patients and carers in the NHS to ensure that their voice is heard and heeded'. (Department of Health 1998)

The many publications that the current Government has published since it came into office indicate that mental health service users have not always received the support and the services that they needed. It is further suggested that for too long people with mental health problems have been stigmatised by society, in communities, in the workplace and in the media and that is why improving mental health services is among the Government's key priorities. Delivering on the standards set out in the National Service Framework are seen as a means to bring about the improvements that people with mental health problems ought to have.

Thus it is clear that the Government has concluded that users' views on their own care and treatment should be sought and that this is intrinsic to achieving quality outcomes within mental health services. The aims of rationalisation and efficiency of the previous Government are retained but firmly welded to this are effective outcomes defined in terms of meeting users' needs. Policy has expressed the logic that working within resources and achieving financial targets is of little use if outcomes are of poor quality and not user focused. However, there is a blot on the collaborative landscape since at present the Mental Health Act 1983 is under review and is due to be reported upon. There is considerable concern being expressed about the nature of the draft Mental Health Bill, in particular the proposals regarding compulsory treatment orders.

Users' views challenge the orthodoxy of what traditionally the system has defined as successful outcomes, which includes a concept of the 'efficient nurse', and has set a new agenda for what nurses need to do, be and know. If the aims of the World Health Organization and the Government are to become a reality within mental health services then a collective user perspective must not only be sought and reflected within nursing and other health care professionals' curricula and practice but also acted upon in practice. Participation is seen as a means of achieving empowerment, which has been defined as 'a process by which individuals gain mastery or control over their own lives and democratic participation in the life of their community' (Zimmerman & Rappaport 1988). Oakley (1989) notes that health professionals, at least in theory, support client participation in their own health care. The NHS (10 year) Plan sets out to transform the health and social care system so that it produces faster, fairer services that deliver better health and tackles health inequalities. Only as the plan unfolds, together with the National Framework for Mental Health, Clinical Governance and other policies, will we be able to see the extent to which user issues have been taken onboard and developed. Partnership, culture, shared values and beliefs are often in a constant state of flux and the values within any organisation are usually expressed through its management and leadership style. This in turn affects the level of commitment from all the players and only when there is some balance between these factors will the agenda for change that reflects a user perspective become a reality.

The key building block to achieving such change has to be made by including the views of service users and involving them in all aspects of their care, from the planning and monitoring of services to the training of staff and the employment of users within mental health services.

SUMMARY

In reflecting on the literature relating to users' perceptions and expectations of nursing care, it is quite clear that the issues of greatest concern tend to be associated with choice, individuality, information, treatment modalities other than drugs, unhelpful and sometimes damaging services and the disregarding of users' experiences. Lack of information is a theme that can be identified throughout, despite the fact that this is recognised by professionals (Islington Mental Health Forum 1989, Rogers et al 1993) and policy makers who acknowledge the need for closer collaboration and participation (Department of Health 1989, 1997).

The types of nursing skills users have indicated are desirable relate to basic support that is given in a sensitive manner when they are distressed. The ability to listen is highly rated. There is more emphasis being given to interpersonal relations and less mention of any structured treatment modalities such as cognitive, behavioural or group therapeutic interventions. Holyoake (1997) indicated that mental health nursing has at the heart of its practice the use of the 'therapeutic self' and if nurse contact and relationship building is central to this practice then much importance must be placed upon actual contact time with users. From the literature reviewed, it appears that nurses do not spend sufficient time with users, despite users expressing views that this is desirable and a means of gaining information and possibly solving problems. Linked to this, a change in attitudes of health care professionals is also being called for in terms of relating to users as 'people' rather than as 'patients'.

The other major issue for users is the importance of the context of their lives relating to loneliness, shortage of money, poor accommodation and the lack of occupation or employment. These factors contribute to their perceptions of being on the margins of society and thus require a clear strategy for intervention and change. Users' medical diagnoses and their mental illness tend to take a back seat to issues relating to everyday living and the isolation that some users experience through stigma, negative assumptions about their capabilities and hence the lack of opportunity to be part of the nation's workforce. Sadly, it also appears that the problem of stigma and prejudice appears to be getting worse not better.

In spite of that, user groups are becoming more organised, articulate and informed and they are keen to develop opportunities for partnership to influence policy, planning and services that reflect their perceived needs based upon their experiences of the current services. If users' views are to be taken seriously it is apparent that what is required is a service that offers choice, genuinely engages in negotiated care and actively promotes the notion of participation, collaboration and partnership.

References

Barker P J, Walters P J 1993 Perceptions of service provision in mental health - a descriptive study of service users and providers. Final report (unpublished). Department of Psychiatry, University of Dundee

Brandon D 1991 Listen to the real experts. Nursing Times 87(49):33

Camden Mental Health Consortium 1988 Treated well? - A code of practice for psychiatric hospitals. Good Practices in Mental Health 5

Campbell P 1996 Working with service users. In: Sandford T, Gournay K (eds) Perspectives in mental health nursing. Bailliere Tindall, London ch 1

Department of Health 1989 Caring for people. HMSO, London

Department of Health 1994 Working in partnership - report of the Mental Health Nursing Review Team. HMSO, London

Department of Health 1998 Press release 98/271:1July

Dodd T 1998 The social construction of the mental health user. Mental Health Practice 8(6):21-25

Essex B, Doig R, Renshaw J 1990 Pilot study of shared care of people with mental illness. British Journal of Medicine 300(6737):1442-1446

Fielding R G, Llewelyn S P 1986 Communication training in nursing may damage your health and enthusiasim: some warnings. Journal of Advanced Nursing 11:529-533

Foucault M 1967 Madness and civilisation. Tavistock, London

Griffiths Report 1983 Recommendations on the effective use of manpower and related resources. HMSO, London

Health Committee Report 1994 First report: better off in the community? The care of people who are seriously mentally ill. HMSO, London

Health Service Commissioner for England, Scotland and Wales 1993 Annual report for 1992-93. HMSO, London

Hogman G, Melzer D 1992 Talk-don't inject. Nursing Times 88(49):61-62

Holloway F 1988 Psychiatric day care. The users' perspective. International Journal of Social Psychiatry 35(3):252-264

Holyoake D 1997 Exploring the nature of nurse interaction using an 'interaction interview schedule'. The results. Psychiatric Care 4(2):83-84

Illich I 1977 Limits to medicine. Penguin, Harmondsworth

Islington Mental Health Forum 1989 Fit for consumption? Mental health users' views of treatment in Islington, London. Islington Mental Health Forum 9

Leary J, Brown D 1995 Findings from the Claybury study of ward based psychiatric nurses and comparisons with community psychiatric nurses. In: Carson J, Fagin L, Ritter S Stress and coping in mental health nursing. Chapman and Hall, London

Lindow V 1990 Participation and power. Openmind 44:10-11

Lindow V 1993 Mental health services. A users' perspective. Communicare. Department of Health, London

McIntyre K, Farrell M, David A 1989 In-patient psychiatric care. The patient's view. British Journal of Medical Psychology 62:249-255

Menzies-Lyth I 1970 The functioning of social systems as a defence against anxiety. Reprinted as Tavistock pamphlet no. 3. The Tavistock Institute of Human Relations, London

Millar P, Rose N 1986 The power of psychiatry. Polity, Cambridge

National Health Service Executive 1996 Patient partnership: building a collaborative strategy. NHS Executive, Leeds

Oakley P 1989 Community involvement in health development. An examination of the critical issues. WHO, Geneva

Offe C 1984 Contradictions of the welfare state. Hutchinson, London

Pembroke L 1991 Surviving psychiatry. Nursing Times 87(49):30-32

Rogers A, Pilgrim D 1991 Pulling down churches: accounting for the British mental health users' movement. Sociology of Health and Illness 13(2):129-148

Rogers A, Pilgrim D, Lacey R 1993 Experiencing psychiatry. Macmillan/MIND, London

Sainsbury Centre for Mental Health 2003 On our own terms. The Sainsbury Centre for Mental Health, London

Sheilds P J, Morrison P, Hart D 1988 Consumer satisfaction on a psychiatric ward. Journal of Advanced Nursing 13:396-400

Shields P 1985 The consumers' view of psychiatry. Hospital Health Services Review May:117-119

Stilwell B 1990 cited. In: Brearley S Patient participation: the literature. Scutari, Harrow, p101

World Health Organization 1986 Targets for health for all: implications for nursing and midwifery. WHO, Geneva

Zimmerman M A, Rappaport J 1988 Citizen participation, perceived control and psychological empowerment. American Journal of Community Psychology 16:725-743

Chapter 4

Partnership

INTRODUCTION

What does partnership in care really mean? The concept of partnership will be explored in this chapter in the context of the preceding chapters. Issues of power and empowerment also have to be examined to establish what changes and developments are necessary for partnership working to become genuine rather than mere rhetoric. The current Government's policies relating to mental health services puts users and partnership centre stage, especially in the context of the need for greater collaboration with users and between health and social services. There are, however, certain contradictions in aspects of their policy, in that there is a tendency to give a higher priority to control, compulsory treatment and public safety. That reflects a willingness to pander to the perception that mental health service users are potentially violent and dangerous, a perception often perpetuated by the popular press. This is not to deny that there are a minority of people who are unfortunately very damaged and disturbed and mental health policy must address that, but issues relating to prejudices and resistance within health care services have to be taken into serious consideration if users' voices are really to be listened to and genuine partnerships developed.

First, it is important to identify exactly what it is that we mean by partnership in care. There are two main themes here: 1) the broader vision in terms of policy development and the integration of services and interprofessional and interagency working to provide 'joined up care' or 'seamless services', to which many of the policy documents frequently refer, and 2) the actual interface between individuals at service delivery level. The former will be discussed but it is the latter that forms the main topic of discussion and concern within this book. Partnership can be regarded as a contractual relationship, an agreement between two or more persons that engage in a particular venture and if it is to be successful then the agenda has to be transparent and respectful of different viewpoints. A question that clearly has to be addressed is to what extent is the user–professional relationship based upon trust and equality, on a human level? It can be argued that a relationship cannot be equal when one person enters into the relationship from a weaker position of need and in distress. There is clearly an imbalance of power between service users and professionals, with the latter being in a position to set agendas and to control the resources and their allocation. There has been an increase in participation by service user representatives; the role often involves attending various meetings. However, at these meetings there is often a single user representative in a room full of experienced professionals, who are familiar with one another and work together on a daily basis. The agenda is likely to have been agreed before they arrive and discussion papers circulated amongst the professionals. In these circumstances the user representative is often an isolated individual with very little influence. Nevertheless, users want to be involved as much as possible as partners in health care decision making that concerns service developments, policy and their individual health care needs, and achievable changes in practice have to start somewhere.

INTERPROFESSIONAL AND INTERAGENCY WORKING

In its Foreword to *Partnership in Action: New Opportunities for Joint Working between Health and Social Services* (Department of Health 1998) the Government aspires to build a modern, dependable health service with patients having fast access to high quality services based on need. It suggests that the current situation is one characterised by fragmentation and bureaucracy and the Government set its sight on changing this situation and building a system of integrated care, based on partnership. The aim is to see health and social services working much more closely together to protect the most vulnerable and those in greatest need, to make partnership working a reality by removing barriers in the existing system, introducing new incentives for joint working and achieving better monitoring of progress towards joint objectives. The result will be a system where the energies of health and social services are not dissipated in unproductive debate on boundaries but one where people's needs are paramount in developing and delivering services. *The National Service Framework for Mental Health* (Department of Health 1999) was also developed to try to bring together service providers from the various agencies, carers and users, to set out standards that should be expected and to promote a user-focused approach rather than a professional-focused one. The way in which people work and the need for integrated working was also reiterated as one of the main concerns within the *National Health Service Plan* (Department of Health 2002). *The NHS Plan* suggests that service users, carers and the public must become genuinely involved in decision making and that staff must work interprofessionally to deliver care that truly reflects the needs of the user in an open and honest culture if the best of health care is to be provided in a caring and safe environment.

Service users and carers have traditionally not been the central focus of care giving but the current agenda does aim to put the user and their significant others first. However, the issue of integrated working has been on the agenda for a long time and can be traced back to the Alma Ata Declaration in 1978 (International Conference on Primary Health Care 1978), which strongly advocated that professionals and the various health and social care agencies must work together more effectively. Pressure for change had also been growing following a number of high profile cases. One of the most well known cases was the murder of Jonathan Zito, who was stabbed to death by Christopher Clunis, who had a diagnosis of schizophrenia, in 1992 at a London underground station. In 1996 Darren Carr, 26, was jailed for the manslaughter of Susan Hearmon and her daughters Kylie, six, and Anne, four, after he set fire to their house in Abingdon in Oxfordshire. Carr had been detained in a psychiatric hospital before the killing but doctors decided he could be discharged. These cases, amongst many others, unfortunately show that integrated care was not there to give the support and care that these individuals required. The inquiries into these cases showed that lack of communication between health, social services and other relevant agencies were key factors that led to the killings.

Similar conclusions were reached by the Bristol Inquiry (Bristol Royal Infirmary Inquiry 2001) that was published in 2001 into the death of children undergoing heart surgery at the Bristol Royal Infirmary between 1984 and 1995. It concluded that around a third of children received less than adequate care and painted a picture of a flawed system of care with poor teamwork between professionals and too much power in too few hands. The report acknowledged that those working with the children were caring and dedicated but some lacked insight and their behaviour was flawed. To a great extent the flaws and failures were within the hospital, its organisation and culture. The management style was said to be punitive and the environment did not make speaking out or openness safe or acceptable. Although the Bristol Inquiry was not a mental health issue, it does serve to show that a particular culture is widespread in the NHS. It is candid in recognising that the changes it envisages will take time as well as resources and that the *NHS Plan* is a ten-year programme. The proposals suggest a need to invest heavily in the workforce and the infrastructure if change towards a modern, user-centred NHS is to occur.

The Victoria Climbie case, of an eight-year-old, who died in February 2000 in London at the hands of her great aunt and her boyfriend, was unfortunately another tragedy and an example of the absence of seamless services and joined-up care. 'Between April 1999 and February

2000, on more than one dozen occasions the relevant services had the opportunity to intervene to protect Victoria Climbie. More than twelve times in ten months they failed to do so. This was not a failing on the part of any one service. It was a failing on the part of every service' (Department of Health 2003a). The Victoria Climbie Inquiry (Department of Health 2003b) endorsed the view that different agencies and professionals were not working effectively together and considered recommendations that would help prevent such a tragedy happening again. The case has highlighted, very tragically, the necessity for professionals and agencies to work together effectively to provide joined-up care, and has been influential in demanding a commitment for them to do so.

Even so, more recently (2003), in the area of mental health services, an investigation has begun into why a person was released from a psychiatric hospital a month before he went on to murder two victims. The BBC reported that the police were not consulted about the decision to allow Anthony Hardy back into the community although the health officials knew he had come under suspicion over the death of a woman whose body had been found in his flat, although it was later confirmed that she died of a heart attack. Marjorie Wallace, Chief Executive of the mental health charity SANE, questioned the decision to release Hardy because he was judged not to pose a risk and stated: 'We are increasingly concerned at the way in which not only families, but others involved in the care of a person discharged from hospital are given partial or no information' (BBC News 2003).

It is the case that cultures that have evolved within organisations over many years can be very difficult to change. The term 'multidisciplinary working' has been prevalent within health and social services for a long time but in practice it tends to translate into different professionals with their own power bases working alongside one another in a hierarchical order that often results in inadequate standards of care and/or mistakes being made since decisions are made with insufficient information and a lack of collaboration. The emphasis upon 'inter' professional and 'inter' agency working suggests that there is a need for individuals to work much more together in a cooperative and collaborative manner with ideas and knowledge being shared and hierarchical authority more receptive to the views of others. Gibbons (1999) describes inter professional working as a deeper level of collaboration in which processes such as evaluation or the development of care plans are done jointly, with professionals of different disciplines putting their knowledge together in an independent manner.

However, Millar (1999) suggests that teams have different ways of working and outlines three distinct behaviours; firstly she describes the fragmented approach. Within this kind of team working there tends not to be any shared vision or philosophy of care, team meetings are rare, communication is poor and problem solving and decision-making tends to be a single professional activity. An understanding of others' roles is absent and professionals are very protective of their boundaries, knowledge and skills. As a result, the service user is lost in a sea of uncertainty. The second style of working is core and peripheral working, whereby there is a core team, perhaps within a hospital, but others are very much on the fringe. A shared vision and philosophy may prevail within the core group but meetings between all concerned parties are rare, communication is mixed and the core group tends to be better informed than the peripheral agencies. Role understanding is seen as superficial and with an absence of any role flexibility. Thirdly, and ideally, what should be happening is integrated working. Integrated working is characterised by a shared philosophy of care and a vision of team working that puts the user at the centre. All team members are not only encouraged but also expected to contribute to the problem solving process. Responsibility is collective, communication meaningful, information and knowledge freely shared. There is understanding and flexibility of roles according to user requirements and a pool of team skills identified to enable joint therapeutic interventions.

There are obvious advantages to the latter way of working: continuity and consistency of care, a possible reduction in ambiguity and effective decision making processes through the sharing of information that draws upon a wider source of ideas. A joint philosophy can lead to a certain team spirit, but this still begs the questions, how do we achieve such effective team working and do we really want to? A team, according to Payne (2000), 'is a group of people each of whom possesses particular expertise; each of whom is responsible for making individual decisions; who together hold a common purpose; who meet together to communicate, collaborate and consolidate knowledge from which plans are made, actions determined and future decisions influenced'. If we are to achieve this then it is important that we understand the dynamics of groups/teams. Tuckman's (1965) 1965 model is still useful and relevant and can help us perhaps to understand and appreciate team development, although there are also many other models of team development. He suggests that there are five stages with each stage having a general theme that describes the group activity.

- Stage 1 – Forming (orientation): The forming stage is regarded as rather superficial with individuals endeavouring to get know one another but at the same time mistrusting and not being sure of each member's ability or agenda. Certain basic ground rules may be established.
- Stage 2 – Storming (conflict): Conflict is not necessary a negative factor, it has an element of sorting out individuals' positions and roles. Alliances may be struck, pairing and subgroups will inevitabley be developed. This stage is more real, with issues of control and power coming into play.
- Stage 3 – Norming (cohesion): A norm is established as to how a particular team will function; individuals' strengths and needs are usually ascertained and a common perspective tends to emerge with a certain amount of emotional attachment amongst team members.
- Stage 4 – Performing (performance): This stage is reached when the team is able to get on with the task in hand and to focus on working towards specific goals rather than looking in at themselves.

- Stage 5 – Mourning (dissolution): Certain individuals will leave the team and new members will arrive. As a result the dynamics will change and often teams revert back to an earlier stage usually characterised by conflict (Stage 2, Storming) until new relationships and perspectives are formed.

A model may be helpful to understand teamworking processes but in practice there are usually other (sometimes more mundane) issues that have to be considered as to why teams don't work. Inevitably there are people who do not even like one another and personality clashes will get in the way. Others will have their own agendas, working at cross purposes to other team members. Uncertainty of roles and people not really knowing what is expected of them, poor or no effective leadership and sticking rigidly to protocols that have long outlived their usefulness are other possible problems. Of course, how effectively teams function will have a direct impact upon how service users' needs are met and power relationships certainly cannot be ignored.

POWER

What is power? Primarily, it is the ability to get others to do what you want them to do, when you want them to do it and in the manner that you expect. The fundamental objective is control. The history of the concept of power is beyond the scope of this chapter but nevertheless in the context of Machiavelli (1469–1527), who wrote about the use of deception and opportunism to manipulate others to achieve certain ends and to maintain power, it is not too difficult to see that his ideas are still relevant and thriving in the 21st century.

The essential ingredient of power can be understood as people's capacity to achieve desired outcomes. The concept is difficult to measure, but has something to do with who wins, who controls the greatest resources and who receives the greatest rewards. Who becomes powerful depends on a number of variables such as knowledge, skills, autonomy, personal qualities, individual drive, culture, authority, expectations and how society perceives certain roles. And of course power can be used both constructively and destructively. Power can also mean the capacity to induce others to do things they would not otherwise have done and there are different ways in which power is exercised, from authority to force. Harrison et al (1992) suggest that there are two main views about the distribution of power in contemporary societies.

In elitism, power is concentrated in the hands of a relatively cohesive few, for example the medical and legal profession. Doctors are powerful collectively at national level and equally powerful at local levels. They control admissions, referrals, discharges, diagnosis and choice of therapy and care. In turn these decisions have resource implications for their own work and the work of other staff, and such decisions are rarely challenged. A client/patient is the client/patient of a named consultant, not of a manager or nurse or social worker, and hence there is authority vested in them. Lukes (1974) raised another aspect of power, which is its relationship to authority. Authority is the right to command or rule some groups of people. It can be attributed either to individuals (the authority of the ward manager or the senior social worker) or to institutions, and varies in its significance (the authority invested in the hospital). Authority, as distinct from power, exists only when those who comply do so because they recognise the legitimacy of the body issuing the command. It thus contrasts both with obtaining compliance by force and with rational persuasion. Authority is a pervasive feature of social life, present in families, schools, businesses, hospitals, social services and churches as well as in the formal apparatus of the state. There are also different types of authority. Weber (Roth & Wittich 1978) in a classic analysis in his work *Economy and Society*, distinguished three basic types: charismatic, the authority of the outstanding individual seen as carrying out a superhuman mission; traditional, the deference shown to those whose right to rule derives from long-established practice (for example the myth that 'doctors know best'); rational–legal, the authority of institutions (Trusts and especially bureaucracies) set up to achieve specific social purposes.

Doctors have a great deal of micro power and are able to maintain their elitist position as they are trained and educated to a high level of expertise and managers cannot replace them with a more compliant group of workers. Power can be diffused more readily within nursing and social work with various care assistants. The medical profession enjoys high social status and respect and most clients/patients want to believe in their extreme skill and ethical commitment. It is not just the general public who accept the authority of doctors but other professionals also defer to their authority. Ward rounds continue to promote the cult of the individual consultant with juniors and nurses in pursuit, the doctor clearly the star. These cultural factors have enabled doctors to maintain their position with the minimum of conflict and many managers have side stepped the issue of doctor power.

The second view of power in contemporary societies is pluralism, a condition in which power is diffused throughout society with no single group controlling all decisions. Power is more widely dispersed among a variety of interest and pressure groups, each of which is able to wield influence in its own particular sphere of decision-making. A pluralist system, as it would apply to the NHS, is one in which decision-making is divided among many independent groups and inter-professional teamwork is an aspiration, as is user empowerment. It is a system where the power of professionals begins to be questioned and it is acknowledged that they do not always know what is best so that users' and carers' views must be taken into consideration when decisions are being made.

Like exponents of elitism, who believe that power is concentrated in the hands of an elite, advocates of pluralism acknowledge that, even in democratic systems, it is a small minority that tends to makes the majority of decisions, but they maintain that no single group should dominate all decisions. They also believe that individuals should have an opportunity to become involved in making decisions, even if they often choose not to do so. The fact that these views, elitism and pluralism, have some plausibility illustrates how difficult it is to find an objective way of measuring power. If we reflect upon the pace of change we see that it is often slow in coming despite the impact of government initiatives and changes in legislation. Management can exercise much power and influence change, but there are limits, and the power of doctors to resist challenges and the entrenchment of traditional ways of doing things are often grossly underestimated.

Power is not only a matter of actuality but also of perception. The corollary of power is dependence and the two are inversely related. Freedom from dependence is autonomy, but we are all dependent to a certain degree and hence autonomy is not an absolute state. As individuals we also have our own self-perception regarding internal/external locus of control and this will affect the way in which we all assert ourselves, contribute to the decision making processes and the degree to which we involve the service users as true partners in care and to which service users involve themselves.

PARTNERSHIP INTERFACE – PERSON–TO–PERSON RELATIONSHIP

Current health care policies continue to put the service user at the centre of their own health care needs. The White Paper, *The New NHS: Modern – Dependable* (Department of Health 1997) favoured a bottom-up approach with public consultation to help empower service users and to move towards partnership working. All care and treatment delivered should be seen as being a partnership with the service user and it is generally accepted that effective partnership will lead to high-quality mental health care. However, from a user perspective how can 'effective partnership' be achieved when a medical model of psychiatry has been used to explain reality and to control and standardise it? As a result, health care systems tend to lead to the disempowerment of users. The current emphasis is that, as far as possible, policies and procedures must be flexible and adaptable to meet the needs of individual service users and to establish meaningful partnership relationships. It is not going to be easy, as many professionals may want to hang on to their positions of power and prestige, and the high salaries that tend to follow.

Nurses could be the key players in promoting partnership working at grass roots level, as they are the people who could spend the greatest amount of time with service users and are the major group in terms of numbers, although it would be naive to believe that nurses could achieve this on their own. Nevertheless, if nurses value their work, themselves and work in a supportive environment then they may be able to play a key role in promoting services that are genuinely user-centred, needs-led and based upon partnership working. Humanistic psychology has had a profound effect upon mental health nursing that is encapsulated in its language of person-centred care and holistic practice and the need for open and honest person-to-person relationships. Egan's (2001) three stage 'Skilled Helper Model' is a useful model in helping people to explore, understand and take more control over their own specific mental health problems and it can provide nurses with an effective tool for working in partnership with users. The goals of using the model are to help people to manage their problems of living more effectively, develop opportunities more fully and to help people become better at helping themselves in their everyday lives. Thus there is an emphasis on empowerment and the person's own agenda is central and the model seeks to move the person towards action leading to outcomes that they choose and value. It is a framework for conceptualising the helping process and is best used in working on issues in the recent past and the present. As with any model, it provides a map, which can be used in exploring and should be used flexibly as a guide, a conceptual framework and not something that must be followed rigidly. Egan's model starts from looking at the 'present scenario' – that is, what is going on now to render an individual dysfunctional? The 'preferred scenario' indicates the changes they really want and a 'strategy for getting there' is based on realistic opportunities and the capability that the individual has.

The idea of emplowerment can mean different things. used as a management buzz word during the 1980s, it subsequently came to be regarded with some cynicism as rhetoric. However, it is significant when its meaning involves the process by which an individual gains feelings of worth, importance and potency. It is about enabling people to take control of their lives and futures and it is important that service providers recognise that users do have certain skills, knowledge and potential and can be trusted to work in partnership in making decisions about their own health care needs. This can lead to users gaining self-confidence and motivation to take control over their lives that they may temporarily have lost. Since many people with a diagnosis of a mental illness have been conditioned by society to feel a level of uneasiness about their condition, their self-esteem is lowered and feelings of powerlessness increased relative to others. However, people who have experienced mental health services do have a viewpoint of that experience, be it positive or negative, and it should be the responsibility of professionals to create an environment in which that knowledge is brought out and used for the benefit of the users and the organisation. Empowerment is an enabling process that removes unnecessary restrictions and moves responsibility back towards the individual. It involves a move from reliance on control to a reliance on partnership working through openness and trust.

Within the context of relationship building, Rogers (1951) spoke about the need for 'core conditions' to prevail with the helpers' approach being based on empathy, warmth and genuineness. Ways of expressing our values are through our behaviour towards others – we have to be available for them and unfortunately research by Gijbels and Burnard (1995), and Edwards (2000), suggests that nurses do not spend sufficient time with users on a one-to-one basis to explore their difficulties or their illness and as a result users' needs are not always understood or met. Empathy is a concept that is spoken about a great deal within mental health services, as if it were a given. As with 'empowerment', words are easily spoken but their meaning can often be lost and they become mere rhetoric. Empathy is about responding in a way that conveys the message that you really understand what it may be like to metaphorically stand in another person's shoes and to appreciate the fit from their perspective; one should try to convey the message that 'I am with you'. Warmth is about valuing users as people and not just as an illness entity, and allowing them to express their personal feelings whatever they may be without judging them or falling into the parent–child relationship. This is far more difficult to achieve in practice as nurses are not always as self-aware as perhaps they should be in developing therapeutic relationships and as a result they can be judgemental and this gets in the way of forming a true partnership working relationship in care. Genuineness is about being with people without judging them, showing that we really care, not being defensive and being able to say what we really think and feel. It is not about hiding behind professional façades or engaging in phoniness, it is about being oneself.

Diagnostic labels can be stigmatising and influence how people are perceived and the degree to which equal relationships can be achieved. A medical diagnosis of 'schizophrenia' often becomes 'schizophrenic' used not as an adjective but as a noun thus reducing the person to an illness entity and underemphasising social, economic and political forces in the determination of ill health. Labels such as 'schizophrenic', 'hypomanic' or 'depressive' are social constructs that tend to devalue the person and often result in a downward spiral of stigma. The person is not seen as normal, and this can lead to rejection, isolation, further loss of personal esteem and a career as a service user dependent upon professionals within mental health/illness services. The media can be outspoken when reporting cases of people with mental health problems and this often reinforces this negative labelling approach. When, in September 2003, boxer Frank Bruno was admitted to a psychiatric hospital, the headline on the front of *The Sun* newspaper was 'Bonkers Bruno locked up'. Such reporting can feed into the public's (and some professionals') imagination, leading to a perception of people with mental health problems as unpredictable and dangerous. The label 'paranoid schizophrenic' can be a real burden for people with a diagnosis of schizophrenia who may be trying to rebuild their lives. It is important that we focus upon users' needs and problems rather than on media or diagnostic labels per se.

Despite a number of NHS reforms and the introduction of the Community Care Act in which service providers are expected to seek users' views, in practice users still do not always feel that they have been heard or listened to. How, then, can working in partnership be achieved? Perhaps the starting point for developing partnership is that service providers/professionals must not only listen to what users are saying but really hear their voices. Providers need to understand what users want, what users see as their needs and priorities and to encourage them to make choices about their treatment and care. The needs and views of users should determine the nature of the service, the care and treatment that is made available to them, and the role of staff should be to facilitate choice and promote self-efficacy as much as this is possible rather than allowing people to slide into a dependency relationship. One important aspect of the process of initiating a partnership is time; time has to be devoted to users before a trusting working relationship can be built. This is not just about ensuring that resources are used to provide that time. As Menzies-Lyth (1970) study suggested, nurses often immerse themselves in tasks that keep them away from service users as a psychological defence mechanism. Time spent with users could result in effective relationships being built and this in turn could result in information and concerns being shared that make the nurse/professional feel uncomfortable and unsure how to respond. To avoid such anxiety it may be easier to spend time in the office doing paper work rather than engaging with users. We look to training to give nurses the skills to form these more intense professional relationships with service users, which must form the basis of true partnerships in care.

When people begin to work together in partnership it is normal to feel anxious, excited, puzzled and sometimes overwhelmed but it is important that we understand one another as individuals with our own idiosyncrasies before we can engage effectively in partnership building. When a person is referred to mental health services they bring with them not only their presenting symptoms of their distress and ill health but also a high degree of anxiety that has to be accommodated. It is essential to spend time at this early stage to begin the building of a therapeutic relationship if a plan of care is to be developed based on working in partnership. The Care Programme Approach (CPA) was introduced in 1991 in an attempt to improve and standardise the delivery of community care services and gave guidance on how they should fulfil their duties as laid out in the NHS and Community Care Act 1990. It hoped to provide a framework for effective mental health care. The CPA is a model for good practice and its four elements are:

1. Systematic arrangements for assessing the health and social needs of people accepted into specialist mental health care services;
2. The formation of a care plan which identifies the health and social needs required from a variety of providers;
3. The appointment of a care coordinator to keep in close touch with the service user and to monitor and coordinate care;
4. Regular reviews and, where necessary, agreed changes to the care plan.

In 2001 an audit pack for monitoring the CPA was introduced (Department of Health 2001). The CPA should govern the care of people but on interviewing twenty-five users in 2003 who had recently been discharged from hospital only nine had a written copy of their care plan, ten were not certain (sic) if they had one or not and only seven stated that they understood the purpose of the CPA. This is rather disconcerting considering that Standard 5 of the *National Service Framework* indicates that each service user should have a copy of a written agreed care plan which sets out the care and rehabilitation to be provided, identifies the care coordinator and specifies the action to be taken in a crisis. If care plans are meant to be an agreement between professionals and the service users then care plans could be a useful tool for fostering partnership working. Sadly some of the users interviewed stated that a care plan was something that the professional did in the office without them being there. This practise obviously needs to change and surely nurses are well placed to transform partnership working from mere rhetoric into effective everyday practise. Formal planned contact that is open and honest with interaction through regular individual sessions and meetings focusing on what users may want to achieve and in a language that partners understand should not be difficult to organise. Successful partnerships start with partnerships between people first and partnerships between organisations are built on that. Users in many ways are experts by experience and if we do not engage effectively with users we will never be able to appreciate their problems and difficulties in the context of their perceptions and lives. An important feature of successful partnerships is that the relationships between the partners are considerate and trustworthy and this cannot be achieved if time is not made available.

The nursing process can be a useful tool for a working partnership relationship and if users are not involved in devising and agreeing their care plan it should come as no surprise to discover that the plan is not being adhered to. Meaningful care plans must involve the user if there is to be a high level of commitment. Partnership working can sometimes be perceived as 'harmonious' but in reality a mature partnership should be able to accommodate differences of opinion, conflict and distrust. It is a common cliché that everyone knows something but no one knows everything. Part of partnership working should be about finding out, understanding and discovering solutions to complex issues. For services to be responsive to the real needs of those that use them then we first have to be aware of what it is that users want from such services. The next chapter reports research findings into users' and nurses' perceptions of the role of the nurse with respect to meeting the needs of users.

References

BBC News 2003 Inquiry into triple killer's care. Online. Available: http:/ / news.bbc.co.uk/1/hi/england/london/3238718.stm

Bristol Royal Infirmary Inquiry 2001 The inquiry into the management of the care of children receiving complex heart surgery at the Bristol Royal Infirmary. Royal Infirmary, Bristol

Department of Health 1997 The new NHS: modern - dependable. The Stationary Office, London

Department of Health 1998 Partnership in action - new opportunities for joint working between health and social services. Department of Health, London

Department of Health 1999 The national service framework for mental health. The Stationary Office, London

Department of Health 2000 The NHS plan. The Stationary Office, London

Department of Health 2001 An audit pack for monitoring the care programme approach. Department of Health, London

Department of Health 2003a Press release. 28th January

Department of Health 2003b The Victoria Climbie inquiry. HMSO, London

Edwards K 2000 Service users and mental health nurses. Journal of Psychiatric and Mental Health Nursing 7: 555-565

Egan G 2001 The skilled helper. Wadsworth, Florence,KY

Gibbons B 1999 An investigation into inter-professional collaboration in stroke rehabilitation team conferences. Journal of Clinical Nursing 8:246-252

Gijbels H, Burnard P 1995 Exploring the skills of mental health nurses. Avebury, Aldershot

Harrison S, Hunter D, Marnoch G, Pollitt C 1992 Just managing: power and culture in the NHS. Macmillan, London

International Conference on Primary Health Care 1978

Declaration of Alma-Ata. Alma-Ata, USSR, 6-12 September

Lukes S 1974 Power: a radical view. Macmillan, London

Menzies-Lyth I 1970 The functioning of social systems as a defence against anxiety. Reprinted as Tavistock pamphlet no. 3. The Tavistock Institute of Human Relations, London

Millar C 1999 Shared learning for pre-qualifying health and social care students: have universities missed the point? Conference paper given at BERA conference, University of Sussex, 3rd September

Payne M 2000 Teamwork in multi-professional care. Macmillan, Basingstoke

Rogers C 1951 Client-centered therapy. Houghton Mufflin, Boston

Roth G, Wittich C (eds) 1978 Max Weber - economy and society. University of California, California

Tuckman B W 1965 Developmental sequences in small groups. Psychological Bulletin 63:384-392

Chapter 5

Users and nursing perceptions

CHAPTER CONTENTS

INTRODUCTION

This chapter draws upon research (Edwards 1999) relating to service user and nursing perspectives with respect to users' needs and the role of the nurse. If effective partnership working relationships are to be established then it is vital that professionals understand what users perceive as their problems, needs, priorities and possible solutions. The methodology that was used in collecting the data is presented, as it is important that there is transparency of the research process to allow others to assess the validity of the findings. Some of the verbatim accounts will be presented, in the belief that this adds to the depth of understanding of the issues of concern from both service users' and nurses' perspectives.

The methodological approach for the study falls into two categories. Firstly, qualitative methods were used for the agenda setting stage by way of Focus Group discussions that allowed respondents to tell their story in their own way and in their own words. Allport (1942) over sixty years ago suggested that if you want to know something about people's activities, then the best way of finding out is to ask them. This maxim is still pertinent today although we have to bear in mind that what people say they do is not always the same as what people may actually do. Secondly as a way of targeting a larger audience, quantitative data collection methods were employed by means of questionnaires. Thus, by combining both qualitative and quantitative methods, it was hoped to bestow a greater understanding, to strengthen and enrich the data gathered. As Jick (1993) suggests, if there is convergence of the data collected by different methods it provides added confidence in the results and even when there is no convergence, explanations can still be generated (although, as White (1990 p9) points out, 'the task of generating data which can claim to represent the views of an entire group is often difficult and sometimes almost an impossible task').

Groups of users of mental health services were contacted and recorded group discussions took place to gain qualitative data about the role of the mental health nurse. Four groups totalling 28 users participated at this stage. Similarly, four groups of mental health nursing students in the final phase of their course, within the last six months, were also contacted for the purpose of setting an agenda on their terms for further investigation. The student numbers totalled 44. This initial stage of the data gathering process was influenced by the principles of the 'Focus Group Interview'. This is a research method that has been used a great deal within marketing research to collect data from consumers in order to provide services that respond to their needs and hence influence the uptake of that particular service. According to Basch (1987) 'the focus group interview is a qualitative research technique used to obtain data about the feelings and opinions of small groups of participants about a given problem, experience, service or other phenomenon'. This method, Basch suggests, is under-utilised within health education and research. Focus group interviews are usually audio taped, transcribed and subjected to an analysis of content that seeks to establish a consensus and generally focuses on description, feelings and problems to be resolved. Findings are not always generalised to larger groups and can be criticised for this, although quantitative techniques are often undertaken as a follow-up study to assess the strength of conviction and the degree to which the findings can be generalised. The use of questionnaires might produce data that can be generalised but they can also be criticised for claiming to represent an accurate or objective measurement of what is often a subjective experience, which actually falls outside the terms of the questionnaire.

The first stage of the data collecting process can be regarded as being influenced by a phenomenological approach, which is said to underpin all qualitative research because it focuses on the individual's interpretation of their own experiences. In setting this research agenda the intention was to discover how both service users and nursing students perceived their world from their subjective experience and what interpretation they brought to bear upon it. A phenomenological approach concerns itself with the meanings, definitions and interpretations that are made by the subjects of the study and has greater potential for depicting their world and priorities more accurately than methods that begin by preconceiving that world and its meaning.

A concern of this research was to avoid the imposition of an agenda that could be regarded as a preconceived professional one. Stevens et al

(1993) draw attention to the importance of phenomenological research methods for nursing, in that 'Practice is a lived experience and as such involves not only the nurse but other health professionals and at the centre the client (the nursed). It involves human beings experiencing and interacting'. One can argue about the semantics of what constitutes a phenomenological approach; however, a premise of this research was that discovering individuals' interpretation of their own experiences can further one's understanding of what caring means to users and nurses and this in turn may lead to influencing how partnership working relationships develop in practice. However, one cannot be complacent in ensuring that the data collection process is reliable and valid.

The primary consideration when deciding on the method or methods that are going to be used in data collection is to ensure that the phenomenon under study can be evaluated as objectively as possible. Reliability is a term that has several meanings but as far as measurement is concerned, an instrument is called reliable if it produces consistent measures from time to time and from measurer to measurer. Validity is the ability of a method, test or instrument to measure what it is designed for, or to be sensitive and specific for the phenomenon under study. Qualitative researchers have tended to combine issues of reliability with those of validity and, according to Powers and Knapp (1990), the idea of consistent measures as an expression of reliability is part of research design, such as testing and documenting the reliability of field notes or informants. Strategies to reduce threats to reliability include using a variety of data sources, verification of data through peer examination or participants' review of findings. Lincoln and Guba (1985) suggest that a study can be judged to be reliable if the reader can follow the decision trail used in the research process and if other researchers, by replicating the study, could draw comparable conclusions. Within phenomenological research, data is collected in a way that pays more attention to the perceptions and meanings placed on events by the research participants. However, a threat to validity may result from the researcher becoming too immersed in the context and subjective state of the respondents. Researchers have to be careful to maintain the distance required to describe or interpret experiences in a meaningful and objective way.

When endeavouring to analyse such data, Morse (1994) suggests that in most types of qualitative analysis there are four stages of data analysis:

1. Comprehending; that is, one seeks to understand the data. The method used for this stage of the study was to adopt a content analysis approach whereby the transcripts of recordings from the Focus Groups were systematically examined line by line to identify key words and phrases that suggested certain themes. The context of the communication process was also considered, to deal with distortions in data collection that can lead from the possibility of a message being transformed when it gets to a recipient. An independent associate was used to examine the data as a means of establishing reliability.

2. Synthesising; the data from each of the four groups was collapsed and integrated and combined with field notes in order to establish the most important issues for further investigation.
3. Theorising; from the first two stages one could begin to build and formulate some understanding of the interrelatedness of the various themes and ideas.
4. Recontextualising; one was then able to reflect upon and understand the data in relation to other situations, for example the findings from the literature review.

Despite these procedures, all analytical techniques will be vulnerable to some random sources of error and issues considered to be important by service providers may not be those which are of most concern to service users. Therefore, an attempt was made to overcome this potential problem and to set an agenda that reflected the issues of greatest importance to both groups.

The initial selection process was to work from MIND's (The mental health charity in England and Wales) list of addresses of groups and organisations relevant to user involvement and from lists of user groups in mental health journals. Groups were randomly identified within different health care areas in order to gain geographical variation. Both unfortunately resulted in a considerable amount of work that rendered little return since some of the groups listed no longer existed, were short term or were made up of just one or two individuals, thus indicating a possible 'time limitedness' of such groups. However, there were some responses and, as a result, the choice of groups was mainly opportunistic in that, as and when user groups did reply affirmatively, requests were made to meet with small groups of approximately 6–12 users. These groups were to discuss the issues that they felt were relevant with regard to the role of the nurse in meeting their mental health care needs.

It became apparent that it was necessary to follow the contacts up quickly because of the transient nature of user groups and the difficulty in obtaining a response. The responses from the groups were not simultaneous and the limited replies meant that only one contact was engaged with at a time. Therefore, groups were self-selecting in that those who were able to make arrangements to meet first were the groups engaged with. It was important not to lose a possible source of data but self-selection can give rise to problems of representation and bias since those that have the greatest grievance against the system may be the keenest to speak out. The opportunistic nature of the selection process also meant that it was not possible to adhere to the initial intent of engaging with groups from different health care areas. Snowball sampling further influenced the selection process in that names of other groups/contacts were offered and pursued. There was very little control over the composition of the groups other than to request a certain number (6–12) for the focus groups. The experience drew to attention the need for future data collection to make tentative links at an early stage with the chosen field of research and to follow it up as quickly as possible. It became apparent that one was working in an area that was transitory and subject to sudden change.

In engaging with the groups, the process adopted was to explain first the purpose and the nature of the research, to ensure that the participants fully understood in what they were being asked to participate. Ethical issues were also considered and participants reassured about confidentiality. Assurance was given that no individual would be identified. This was a concern that some users had raised. They were concerned that anything that they narrated would not be reported or commented upon in a recognisable manner, which, they felt, may affect their position as service users adversely in a service upon which they were still very much dependent. The compositions of the different groups were also self-selecting in that users chose to opt in to the research project; there was no attempt to control the configuration of the groups in terms of diagnosis, gender or age. The groups were diverse in their composition but no record was kept of their personal details. The inclusion criteria for users were that they had either been users or were still using mental health services and had received a notable amount of contact with mental health nurses. The participants were informed that the length of the group discussion would be approximately one hour and with permission the discussions would be audio taped and the recordings transcribed. Ethical issues regarding individual consent, confidentiality and anonymity were repeated and emphasised in each group.

Feldman's (1995) experience of data collection suggests that clusters of data tend to stick together, although for this research it was felt that boundaries had to be imposed by way of three questions to keep the discussions within a manageable framework. The main theme that was explored with the user groups focused on the following: What are the views and perceived needs of users of mental health services in the context of the role that users see nurses fulfilling? The discussions were semi-structured with an attempt being made to keep the discourse in the context of the following question: From a user/client perspective, what does a nurse need to do, be and know? Keeping the group focused is an important variable and as Nyswander (1982 p117) concludes, 'if a group is unclear about its objectives there is a danger that a group will not become cohesive, will be insecure, unproductive and perhaps meaningless. Uncertainty of the goal could also result in the group feeling threatened and tensions aroused, released in unproductive ways that is counter-productive to the research process'. In some instances, while meeting with the user groups, the researcher was initially viewed with suspicion; was he another 'professional' jumping on the user development bandwagon to further his own ends at the expense of users of mental health services? This was resolved by clearly explaining the nature of the research in the same vein that Basch (1987 p416) suggests: 'clarifying goals does not necessarily mean revealing the research hypothesis or questions under study. Clarifying goals does mean communicating to participants what you want to know from them'. The repeated reassurance of confidentiality and the answering of their questions were also addressed. All interviews took place in an environment with which the groups were familiar but which was unfamiliar to the researcher, in an attempt to neutralise any imagined or real unequal power relationship. Skills were required in effectively facilitating group functioning and establishing psychological safety to promote a conducive climate in which people could freely and openly express their thoughts and feelings. The audio taped discussions revealed that there were many different views and disagreements rather than a homogenous response that could have given rise to the charge that user groups tend to reflect a particular 'party line'. Neither did the user's state of mind appear to be a problem as it is sometimes assumed when users' views are sought. Folch-Lyon and Trost (1981) maintain that:

'The group situation may also encourage participants to disclose behaviour and attitudes that they might not consciously reveal in an individual interview situation. This occurs because participants often feel more comfortable and secure in the company of people who share similar opinions, attitudes and behaviour or simply because they become carried away with the discussions in the presence of others with similar problems. Given the proper environment participants are less on guard against personal disclosures because the atmosphere is tolerant, friendly and permissive even when selfish, egocentric, aggressive, daring or questionable judgements are voiced'.

Immediately after each group meeting field-notes were made to capture comments and observations that appeared relevant and that had not been recorded by audiotape.

The same methodological approach was applied to mental health nursing students nearing completion of their courses to ascertain how they perceive their future role given that they would be the 'new' generation of mental health nurses. The inclusion criteria were restricted to those who were in the final phase of their course, that is within six months of completion and, as with the user groups, there was no attempt made to control the composition of the nursing student groups with respect to gender or age. There were no significant methodological problems to overcome while meeting with the student groups other than those that have been previously mentioned in relation to the problems of adopting a phenomenological approach and to the problems that would equally apply to user groups.

The *Nursing Applicant Handbook* was used as a source of information about courses and hence as a way of targeting nursing students. Initially it was intended to randomly target one college/university in different parts of the country. Letters were sent to the various Schools/Departments of Nursing but this did prove to be slightly problematic as there were some difficulties in identifying the appropriate person responsible for gaining access. Some tutors and lecturers were uncertain of their authority in putting forward the proposal to the students for them to choose whether or not to participate in the research. The tutors' response to the proposal reflected a need to push the researcher's request up the hierarchy. This may suggest a dependency culture that is still within nursing rather than an autonomous professional one.

Responses from colleges and universities were not simultaneous and those that responded earliest were followed up swiftly with the researcher travelling to the various institutions to meet with the students for the focus group discussions that all took place within their environments. Hence the principle of opportunistic sampling was again adopted in the selection of Schools/Departments of Nursing that were considered to be representative of different parts of the country. There had initially been eight responses but some of these contacts were very slow in offering a positive reply to participate in the research. The decision was made to restrict the number of groups to four because only recurrence of data already discovered was being yielded after meeting with the third group. The fourth group tended to reflect a saturation point. The main perspective focused upon with the student groups was on a similar theme to that which was explored with the user groups. The discussions were semi-structured and there was an attempt to focus and to stick within the boundary of the following question, the same as that put to the user groups: From a student/future nurse perspective what does a nurse need to do, be and know? They were also asked how, as future nurses, they perceived their role given the change in nurse preparation.

Having completed the group discussions with both users and student nurses, the recordings were transcribed and the data analysed in the context of the three questions previously mentioned: What should a nurse do, be and know? The method of data analysis influenced by the ideas of Glaser and Strauss (1967, 1968), Taylor and Bogdan (1984) and Burnard (1991), is described as thematic content analysis. The aim of this approach was to describe, interpret and give meaning to the content and to try and understand what was expected from nursing in the context of users' expressed needs. Glaser and Strauss (1968) adopted 'grounded theory' as an approach to the handling of qualitative data and to the formulation of theoretical propositions. By this term they meant 'the discovery of theory from data' and suggested that such an approach seemed likely to increase the production of research that is detailed, non-trivial and of use to the layperson as well as to the professional. They outline nine stages in handling data, which were used as a framework for analysing the data collected from the Focus Groups for this research:

1. Develop categories
2. Saturate categories
3. Abstract definitions
4. Use the definitions
5. Exploit categories fully
6. Note, develop and follow up links between the categories
7. Consider the conditions under which the links hold
8. Make connections where relevant to existing theory
9. Use extreme comparisons to the maximum to test emerging relationships

According to Turner (1981) the advantages for the researcher in using grounded theory are many. It promotes the development of theoretical accounts and explanations, which conform closely to the situations being observed so that the theory is likely to be intelligible to, and usable by, those in the situations studied. The theories developed are likely to be complex rather than oversimplified ways of accounting for a complex world and it is important to realise that the grounded theorist is not able to mask poor quality work behind an array of impressive techniques, for what he is doing is very much open to scrutiny. In agreement with Turner (1981) 'the process of research should be as open as possible, so that neither the processes of research nor their findings are subjected to mystifications which conceal their true nature from other researchers, from the subjects of research, or from those seeking to understand the research findings when they are reported'. The key issues, various ideas and suggestions that were identified from the Focus Groups were synthesised into themes and subjected to a Rank Order Exercise and the findings were then incorporated into the construction of questionnaires.

A Rank Order Exercise was carried out in an attempt to be more focused and ascertain more specifically the importance attached to the identified issues as to what a nurse should 'do', 'be', and 'know'. A 10% sample as suggested by Oppenheim (1992) of the proposed target population of 400 for Stage 2 (questionnaires) was decided upon. Groups of both users (40) and nursing students (40) were then contacted and arrangements made to meet with the groups. These were different groups to the participants in the Focus Groups but the same method of contact was used. Participants were asked to identify five issues in order of importance to them as individuals. The responses were then compared in an endeavour to distinguish core concerns for users and nursing students and to establish the degree of convergence or divergence at that particular stage of the research. The following are the results of the first stage of the qualitative data collection commencing with the Focus Groups and then the Rank Order Exercise. In presenting the findings no attempt has been made to analyse the data from a particular theoretical perspective. The intention was to describe, interpret and to give meaning to the content and to try to understand the perceptions of the respondents.

FOCUS GROUPS FINDINGS

Having completed the Focus Group discussions and transcribed the recordings the data was analysed in the context of the three questions previously mentioned. That is, what should a mental health nurse do, be and know. An inventory of the identified issues are presented, firstly the issues categorised from the individual groups and secondly synthesised to reflect the integrated view of the four groups of both users and students. The process of achieving this followed the procedure of integrating and/or eliminating recurring issues and the issues are not rank ordered at this stage. The following are the themes that emerged from the Focus Groups.

User groups

Group 1 (8 participants)

- Improved user–nurse ratio, especially at night
- Show respect and a genuine interest
- Traits such as kindness, gentleness and sensitivity
- Treat as an individual and show tolerance
- Time to talk and explore difficulties
- Regularity, consistency and availability of nurses
- Have a genuine interest in mental health nursing rather than it merely being a job
- Life experience and older nurses with maturity
- Exercises and relaxation to music
- Social skills and help in developing a support network
- Nutrition and a good diet
- Information about medication
- Nurses to have insight and understanding of themselves.

The general attitude of the users who participated in this first group meeting appeared to be curious yet positive about being asked to define what they thought the role of the nurse should be. Sadly, the above issues were mentioned as desirable attributes but the group's experiences generally seemed to be negative, characterised by comments such as:

> 'When I was in one hospital the nurses were absolutely unsuited to treat people with mental illnesses. I will give you one example of what happened to me. They would come up to you when you were in bed and say; 'Come on, you are going to have a bath' and they would run the bath, make you get into it and they would just leave you. Then they would come back and throw some clothes that they had got from somewhere. Then they would be shouting; "Have you not finished in there yet?" It took me a long time to enjoy a bath again after that experience.'

This may sound like a description of practices that were part of the culture of the large Victorian institutions but in fact relates to an admission of a 42-year-old woman to a psychiatric wing of a general hospital in the 1990s. It is an example of one of the themes that emerged regarding 'showing respect and a genuine interest'. Other remarks from users were.

> 'Most of the time that I was in hospital therapy was a dirty word, every morning once the tea trolley had been round a nurse would come out shouting, come on, come on, down to therapy which consisted of some useless occupational therapy activity. The same old routine, day in day out.'

> 'The nurses that are sent to the Day Centre at least talk to you there.'

'The nurses that you need to feel the fear from are the regular ones.'

'Mental health is a very low priority in the order of things, the lowest really. The only lower are dead people.'

Group 2 (6 participants)

- Nurses should be informal, friendly and approachable
- Reassuring, give attention and take clients seriously
- Show respect and be able to empathise
- Have time to sit down and just listen (listening skills)
- Help reduce stigma by not labelling and reducing users to mere illness entities
- Facilitate an understanding of situations
- Higher staff/user ratio
- Tolerant, non-threatening
- Counselling skills
- Show affection and warmth
- A sympathetic and safe atmosphere in hospital
- Nurses to explain the effects of drugs and give more information
- Practical help/social skills
- Friendliness and compassionate.

This second group was relaxed and welcoming and at ease in offering their views of the experiences that they had received as users of mental health services. Again, the following comments are examples of what was said by members of the group:

'Firstly someone that will reach out to you because you are in distress and you want a friendly handshake. Hello, hi, just keep it informal because when you are in a state of breakdown or what they call schizophrenia your um, um, probably crying for help and need people to reach out to you in a friendly way, first names, a cup of tea, offer you something because you want help.'

'Things have changed now for the better, clinical coldness when I was first in hospital in 1987. No one reached out to me, it was as if I was there as a punishment.'

'I think an analogy with prison is ... it is a bit, even these days you still feel that way to a certain extent even though there are not too many locks and keys in most psychiatric units, there is still ... control.'

'It's a feeling that, true or not that you are always being watched. I think, a feeling that you are being monitored, being monitored and observed. You feel that you are in a zoo sometimes.'

'I do agree that anyone who needs attention should get the attention. Do you know what I mean? It would stop these attacks coming on so often.'

'The only experience that I have had of a psychiatric unit was that they seemed to be very professional, extremely professional, but on the other hand there did not appear to be many emotions involved.'

On a more positive note:

'One time I can remember in particular when nursing staff did do it very well. At times we have all been prescribed 'as and when necessary' medication, tranquillisers and whatever, and I said; 'Listen, I need this tablet, I am wound up' and she said; 'Right, come in here and sit down', talked with me and that really is what you want. You need more time.'

Group 3 (6 participants)
- Approachable and relate to you as an individual
- Communicate/talk to you and give you feedback
- Give out the drugs
- Need to understand our difficulties, provide company and calmness
- Keep the peace and enforce the rules
- Humaneness
- Advocate
- Structured interaction and need to be competent in therapies
- Older and more mature and more knowledgeable
- Need to do more than simply befriending and reassuring
- Improved personal conduct.

The third group of users were attending a day centre and initially appeared a little suspicious of the researcher's intent, but nevertheless engaged effectively in the discussion.

Some members were very thoughtful in their responses and two made it very clear that they had been diagnosed as suffering from schizophrenia. It was as if this somehow gave them a certain status and added credibility to their views. At the time of the meeting there did not appear to be anything to suggest that a diagnosis of schizophrenia was affecting their ability to contribute effectively to the discussion. It seemed difficult for the group to identify what it was that nurses actually do as the following quotes suggest:

'Well these are not things that I have thought about before but, just off the top of my head, when in hospital occasionally at least they did something valuable by simply being, um ... relating to you and that was generally by having exchanges with other people and you can learn from that.'

'Well, they talk to you.'

'They should be trained to relate to all kinds of people from different occupations, but I just found it difficult to be with them.'

'All they really have to do in a mental hospital is dish out the drugs.'

Another comment describes the experience of a user trying to get a light for a cigarette in a psychiatric hospital as being rather harrowing:

'The whole thing about getting a light if you are a smoker and it could mean a great deal, was the unnecessary daily drama and you thanked your lucky stars if it was as simply as it should be; Just excuse me nurse can I have a light? Yes, sure, no problem. But no it was a constant pressure and drama, just the damn business of getting a light for a cigarette. One did not know if it was a conscious part of a regime of confrontation, disempowering and belittling and sort of controlling patients, or simply neglect and laziness in their responsibilities. It was certainly not about health promotion.'

Group 4 (8 participants)

- More time to talk and build up your confidence
- Help with personal hygiene and provide a safe environment
- More activities and facilitate the expression of feelings
- Talking therapy, listen, observe and promote independence
- Supervise discharge and support in the community
- Should be friendly and take an interest
- Administer medication
- Treat users as human beings and empathise
- Should be there for users and not for the psychiatrist
- Information about medication
- Take users seriously
- Give out food and put people to bed
- More nurses and not abuse authority.

This group discussion took place at a drop-in centre that was user led, with decisions being taken through a committee and consultation with any users there at any particular time. The users responded to the request to participate in the research positively as they felt that they should make use of the opportunity to have their views heard and recorded in the hope that it may influence changes in the psychiatric system. This group entered into a lively, thoughtful and sincere discussion and their responses reflected a range of experiences and conditions extending from admissions for attempted suicide, to being diagnosed as suffering from schizophrenia, mania and depression. Some of the views and feelings are reflected in the following remarks from the recorded discussions:

'I always felt that when I went to the nurse in the office she always told me to go away and come back later. So I kept coming back later and later and it was the same thing. They are so busy that they do not have time for you as an individual.'

The previous and the following quotes are interesting in that the users are showing sensitivity and making allowances for the nurses despite not appearing to get their own needs met:

'I do think that Community Psychiatric Nurses (CPNs) are better than the nurses in hospital because they actually see you, they visit you and they talk to you, whereas in hospital they cannot do that, they have too much to do, they are overworked some of them.'

'The only good thing that happened to me was the student nurses because they actually took time out to listen to you and to do things for you. They are just there to observe or whatever and to learn but I found they were always there to talk to, the student nurses I found most helpful.'

'I think that there is not enough therapy and not enough therapists and we do not need pills all the time. Somebody goes to hospital and they have just lost their husband or their wife, or whatever the case may be and they are suffering from grief and under great stress. Instead of being dished out a dose of tranquillisers or whatever when all they really need is someone to express their grief to. To be able to talk it out, to talk it through, and that is why I think we need more therapists, especially with this community care.'

Synthesis   Having completed the preliminary stage in gaining qualitative data, the data from the four groups of users was combined and then used to devise the questionnaire for the second stage i.e. quantitative data collection. The following data is a synthesis of user views with respect to the question: from a user/client perspective what does a nurse need to do, be and know?

Do?
- Build up your confidence and independence
- Promote meaningful activities
- Treat as an individual and give affection and warmth
- Show respect and a genuine interest
- Give time to talk and explore difficulties
- Show insight and understanding
- Improve user/nurse ratio
- Promote social skills and develop support networks
- Provide a sympathetic atmosphere in hospital
- Give attention and take users seriously
- Help reduce stigma and promote understanding of mental illness
- Provide structure and safety
- Help with personal hygiene
- Listen more and observe
- Follow up community support
- Administer and give information about medication.

Be?
- Consistent, approachable and available
- Nurses in a career not 'just in a job'
- Experience of life, older and mature
- Sensitive, self aware, kind and tolerant
- Non-threatening
- Friendly, human and be able to empathise
- More knowledgeable

- Competent in therapies
- Advocates
- Genuinely interested in people.

Know?
- About medication and its effects (intended and unintended)
- Counselling skills
- About medical and physical problems
- Communication skills
- Talking therapies
- Themselves.

In targeting the user groups an initial concern had been, would the views and information gleaned be that of a 'rehearsed position' and therefore how representative would the views expressed be? This was not the case. In the four groups targeted there was much discussion and healthy rapport, with individuals' views being respected and accommodated despite differences of opinion. It is also noteworthy that on several occasions, when discussing this research with others in the field, the researcher was asked how representative the users were. However, on no occasion was he asked about the representative status of the nursing participants and whether or not they may project a rehearsed position. Epstein and Olsen (1999) also reported that the issue of representativeness is raised whenever users speak out. Furthermore they suggest that 'sometimes, the issue of who is being represented is raised by providers and others, in order to denigrate the arguments of articulate or impassioned users'. Nevertheless, it is important to endeavour to try to know how representative and typical responses are if true partnership working is to prevail.

Student groups

It was easier, despite a few previously mentioned problems, to gain access to student groups due to the co-operation of nurse tutors/lecturers who viewed the research as being of equal concern to them and the students seemed eager in having the opportunity to share their views on how they perceived their preparation and future role. The key issues that emerged from the discussions are as follows:

Group 1 (4 participants)
- Running groups (social skills, reminiscence and relaxation)
- Some teaching and managerial work
- Observing, monitoring and containment of patients
- Socialising to promote social skills, knowledge of social work and occupational therapy
- Role very broad and to do what others do not do
- Sit down and talk, have good interpersonal and counselling skills
- Treat users as individuals, motivate and spend more time with people
- Need to have specialised skills and knowledge
- Manage aggression, diffuse situations and promote safety
- Help work out people's difficulties and devise strategies for coping
- Sensitivity, confidence, more autonomy and power
- Advocate and introduce new ideas and change
- Own life needs to be fairly stable

- Being professional, taking a pride in your work, believing in it and standing up for it
- A need for supervision structures
- Keeping up to date with developments and knowledge
- Greater medical understanding
- Interventions should be theory and research based.

Unfortunately only four student nurses turned up, but nevertheless this first group was articulate and reflective, and the following comments help bring alive some of their views. It was interesting to hear that they saw themselves as being generic in their roles, but the genericism was expressed in the context of social work and occupational therapy rather than reflecting any identification with their peers on other branches of the nursing course, that is paediatrics or 'adult' nursing. The title 'adult nursing', as confirmed by both the ENB and the UKCC, was regarded by the group as serving to alienate those with mental health problems and potential mental health branch students since it infers that mental health services have different service users other than bona fide 'adults'. Altschul (1997) is also of the opinion that psychiatric nurses have more in common with social workers, occupational therapists, counsellors, the police and even prison workers than with general ('adult') nurses. The following are examples of comments that were made:

'The nurses on the wards pick up the bits that other people do not do really; they very much take on a social work role, do some work which traditional occupational therapists would do and very much administrative and managerial work as well. I was a bit disappointed by how little individual work they do with patients and they would not set time aside specifically to see anyone. It was somewhat ... on the run.'

This comment also suggests a theme that emerged frequently whilst engaging with the different groups; that is, the importance of having time to relate to and be with users. Commenting on the importance of this theme the following quotes serve to illustrate the point:

'For me one of the most important things is to spend time with people and see them as individuals and not just as part of the system, but it is hard to do.'

'I think there are skills of being able to take the heat out of situations, being able to make the other patients on the ward feel safe as well as keeping things on an even level; not letting things get out of hand.'

'What can I do? I think it is those interpersonal skills initially. I think we are fairly good at that now and able to suss out what is happening to someone fairly quickly, to pick up on what is going on and what they are feeling and maybe know what to do once we are aware of that. I think that the counselling and therapy skills we are getting are fairly good for this stage, just qualifying, and I think that is quite unusual. Most of the nurses that I have met do not have such a range of skills that we have picked up.'

In relation to change, a student remarked:

'I think many nurses feel threatened by new ideas because it is almost that you are saying, what you are doing is not right. You get so many excuses why something will not work. Some people do not like change, they like the system just as it is.'

Group 2 (18 participants)
- Reduce the stigma associated with mental ill health and help change the image of the service
- Treat users as individuals and human beings
- Communication skills and a good observer
- Be able to facilitate not just control
- Enable users to become more autonomous
- Empower people, not control and institutionalise
- Motivate and enhance their self-esteem
- Promote health education
- Restrain disturbed behaviour
- Theory to inform practice
- A nurse should have maturity and life experience
- Problem solving skills
- Deconstruct our perceptions and reconstruct them from users' views
- A need to question old practices
- Self-awareness, empathy and counselling skills
- Knowledge of general and physical problems.

In the second group, there were eighteen students who were waiting and prepared to participate in the discussion, a much larger group than anticipated. The choice was whether to use certain criteria to reduce the size or to work with the group as it was. The latter course of action was chosen with firm facilitation to ensure effective dialogue of all members and the recording of the discussion.

A great deal of reflection on their course took place within this group and the main feelings that were being expressed were ambivalent ones. They felt that they were being exposed and introduced to relevant information and skills, but there was a concern that they were being disadvantaged by the course, which they perceived as being too 'general nursing' in orientation. There was also concern expressed that there was much pressure to conform to the culture of the environment where they were gaining their clinical experiences and they were experiencing a great deal of cognitive dissonance. They were being exposed to practices that contradicted what they were being taught. It is difficult to predict how this can be resolved, as it has been an issue within nursing for a long time and often referred to as the 'service–education' split. Osgood and Tannenbaum's (1955) congruity theory suggests that the way that cognitive dissonance is resolved is by the individual disregarding the attitude that is held less firmly in order to regain a state of harmony. The following quotes from these students reflect some of their sentiments:

'You are constrained by the ethical and holistic approach that you are supposed to deliver because you are working in a service that has goals that you yourself do not agree with, and you have to live in the real world don't you? We talk about family therapy and behavioural approaches and all the rest of it and ultimately if the medical model does not agree with that method or you yourself have not been trained in it then it will not get delivered. So where are you being the patient's advocate?'

'Why not question what we are looking at, not what you are looking for, and question what you see? I think that is what we are being trained to do, to question what we see. We are looking at research for everything, why this and why that? We are being taught to question everything and if you are told what to look for you will not question anything.'

'It's about empowering people because it's giving power back and it's giving them control. What I have seen in the past has been control by professionals; it's giving choice back. I do not know, but the difference is in the future and not what I have seen in the past.'

'I think you partly empower by not taking on everything that the patient can do for themselves, just the deficits in their abilities. I agree that you empower rather than take away, the nursing profession used to take away much ability that people still had.'

'I feel this training has brought more out of me and I have found out more about myself than anything.'

'By the nature of the job ultimately you are expected to achieve empathy, engage in a counselling process and help reconstruct what the patient is experiencing.'

The above comments provide insight into students' perceptions of their work; they suggest a very thoughtful and real understanding of some pertinent issues facing mental health services. It raises important concerns about what support systems will be in place for newly qualifying nurses to ensure that such insight and enthusiasm is not stifled and lost. That point was one that also emerged in the following group.

Group 3 (11 participants)

- Power so as to be able to influence decisions and make changes
- Be autonomous practitioners with a research knowledge base
- Spend more time with the patients
- Structured and organised activities
- Give out medication
- Paper work/report writing

- Counselling skills
- Advocate and improve relationships with patients
- A need to be proactive
- Topical theory and knowledge base
- More peer support and supervision
- Appropriate financial rewards
- Empower patients
- Health promotion and preventative work in the community
- Improved staff/user ratio
- Provide better leadership and competent specialised nurses
- Become more involved with therapeutic group work.

This group appeared to be genuinely and extremely concerned about the quality of the service that was being provided. They were equally concerned about how they would fit into the scheme of things having been the recipients of a current higher education and training programme that was quite different to the training of the majority of those with whom they had clinical contact. They expressed a fear of being marginalised and having to surrender their convictions and adapt to a long-established way of doing things that was not in keeping with their knowledge and understanding. They also perceived a danger of becoming institutionalised. Their sentiments can be better understood by some of the verbatim comments that were made, for example:

'Someone said something to me the other day they said; "You will not make a good psychiatric nurse because you are too polite to the patients". I thought that was a very interesting comment.'

'I think that if you are abrupt to patients and rude it just reinforces the feeling of failure, it's so sad.'

'Primary nursing is used but it's more abused than used. You are allocated patients on one of those notice boards and it all looks very nice and you ask staff nurses if they have spoken or interacted or done anything with their patients and the answer is invariably they have not.'

On a more positive note:

'I think that you can make a difference when you are there, you can show by example and it does rub off a bit. I think if you persevere and say this is the way I do it, the proper way, it does rub off.'

Group 4 (11 participants) The major concerns expressed by the fourth group were the difficulties in being innovative and in initiating change.

- Empower users by developing and promoting their personal resources
- Individualise care
- Need for appropriate staffing levels
- Managerial role and paper work

- Listen to what the users say and promote new ideas
- Better-educated nurses with more knowledge and research awareness
- Respect for self and others and have a caring personality
- Interpersonal skills to establish therapeutic relationships and the ability to motivate others
- Supervision of practice
- Aware of social needs and information to promote informed decision-making
- More power to empower others and be a person first then a nurse
- Facilitate insight into difficulties
- Help to reduce stigma
- Involve family and significant others
- Promote a partnership in care.

The students in this group expressed a realistic concern as to the power of the status quo and the way in which, on qualifying, they felt that they would no longer have the support and supervision that they had received while on the course. Consequently, there was a fear that they would have to compromise their values and beliefs. Some of students verbatim responses again illustrate these concerns:

'Especially as a student I think there is that pressure to conform to a certain student role. However, on this course I think that is changing a bit because you are encouraged to be more independently minded and question, but the pressure is still there to a certain extent.'

'The wards are dominated by the medical staff so nursing is shoved to the back. The mental health nurse is shoved to the back anyway, in nursing as a whole it is seen as a sub branch and also by the general public. It is an uphill battle.'

'If we do not have the power we can not empower.'

'Nurses are at each other's throats at the moment, they are so dysfunctional. On the last two wards that I have been on it has been like that, so here I am thinking every time I get to work in a team it is when I am in this group. You get feedback, support, discuss issues and I feel that is what I should be getting on the wards. I feel that I have got many skills since starting the course and there are people out there who have been there for years and I do not know what they have done. It is frightening really.'

The following data is a synthesis of student's views on the question: From a student/future nurse perspective, what does a nurse need to do, be and know?

Do?

- Give information
- Facilitate group work and promote social skills
- Observe and monitor and contain patients

- Counselling
- Manage aggression
- Promote a positive image of mental illness
- Spend more time with people
- Treat as individuals and listen to service users
- Motivate others
- Administer medication
- Involve family and/or significant others
- Improve staff/user ratio.

Be?
- Mature and self aware
- Better educated, sensitive and approachable
- Caring, confident and competent
- Specialists
- Autonomous practitioners and more powerful
- Advocates and agents of change
- Proactive
- Better financially rewarded
- Person first then a nurse.

Know?
- Theory and research
- About different life experiences
- More about general and physical problems
- Aspects of social work and occupational therapy
- Communication skills and problem solving approaches
- Keep up-to-date with knowledge and developments.

This initial data reflected some of the issues that were identified by Rogers and Pilgrim (1994) in their survey that involved 516 mental health service users and in a similar vein the responses were based on personal experiences with users expressing comparable views relating to nurses. For example they identified issues relating to interpersonal skills, physical needs, respect and a need to be related to on an ordinary everyday level as opposed to a professional/patient one that tends to reduce them to an illness entity. Those were all issues about which the groups of students and users who were interviewed for this research expressed concern. From the following collation of the synthesised data from both users and student nurses in response to the three key questions, one can identify the convergence of views. There were also issues raised that are of a divergent interest and nature. Firstly, by looking at the response to what nurses should 'do' one can see the commonality and convergence of perceptions (Table 5.1).

Other issues identified by the students that were not mentioned as frequently by users were managing aggression, counselling, administering and monitoring medication. Some of these issues were identified tangentially by some users. For example, time to talk could be seen as being integral to counselling, and providing structure and safety could be central to managing aggression, especially as some users commented in a rather derogatory manner about 'dishing out the drugs'. Issues to which users gave greater emphasis than had nurses

Table 5.1 User and students' perceptions of what a nurse should 'do'

Users' perceptions	Student perceptions
Promote activities	Facilitate group work
Treat as individuals	Treat as individuals
Listen to users	Listen to users
Enhance user confidence	Motivate
Improve nurse/user ratio	Improve nurse/user ratio
Give information	Give information
More time to talk	Spend more time with users
Develop a support network	Involve family and/or others
Reduce stigma	Promote a positive image of mental illness
Social skills training	Social skills training
Promote structure and safety	Contain users

could be regarded as 'matters of integrity'. Those issues were that nurses should show genuine interest, respect, affection and warmth, show insight and understanding, provide a sympathetic atmosphere, help with personal hygiene and follow up with community support. The collated data on what a nurse should 'be' can be seen in Table 5.2.

Again one can see the common ground with respect to what a nurse should 'be' but there are issues on which views between the two groups diverge. These issues, fundamentally, and not surprisingly, reflect a different focus; the organisational perspective of the nurse striving to be part of a professional group and the concerns of users focusing on their relationship with the individual nurse and the effect that nursing practice can have on them. The students' perceptions were that they should be specialists, autonomous practitioners, have more pay and power, be assertive and proactive. Issues identified by users concerned nurses being available, non-threatening, consistent, and showing attitudes that are compatible with a genuine interest in pursuing nursing as a career rather than it being 'just a job'.

Table 5.3 shows the convergent views of the groups about what a nurse should know. For the users, knowledge of medication and its effects was what they wanted information about; the issue emerged as a significant part of their experience as users of mental health services. The students were concerned with issues such as theory and research,

Table 5.2 User and students' perceptions of what a nurse should 'be'

Users' perception	Student perception
Self aware	Self aware
Mature	Mature
Better educated	More knowledgeable
Sensitive	Sensitive and approachable
Competent	Competent
Advocate	Advocates/change agents
Caring	Caring
Friendly and human	Person first then a nurse

Table 5.3 User and students' perceptions of what a nurse should 'know'

Users' perception	Student perception
Medical and physical disorders	Medical and physical disorders
Communication skills	Communication skills
Know themselves	Know themselves
Talking therapies	Talking therapies

problem solving approaches, life experience and aspects of social work and occupational therapy. The issue of counselling was not identified as such by users when asked what nurses should do, but it was mentioned in the context of nurses' knowledge. There may be a question here of whether nurses are dabbling in interventions without having sufficient preparation and training. Counselling and Cognitive Behaviour Therapy appear to be 'band wagons' in nursing at present and, like 'nursing models', taken on board without sufficient digestion. The key concern that users identified was not nurses' skills per se or a need for any specific therapy but that nurses should have the intangible qualities, which could be regarded as integrity and compassion. That issue was identified as long ago as the mid 18th century. Nolan (1993) suggests that William Battie (1703–1776), a pioneer in the care of mental patients, 'was probably the first public figure to recognise the importance of a compassionate personality when caring for the insane; it was his observation that some patients, treated only with kindness and decency, made full recoveries despite lack of access to any recognised treatment. Kindly carers and a calm environment were prerequisites if any treatment regimen was to be effective'. It is also noteworthy that the response to the question 'what should nurses know?' had the least amount of content to its answer. These initial findings are encouraging in that the expressed views of both users and students are generally convergent but it also begs the question, will they remain so in actual practice?

Rank order exercise

The convergent and divergent issues were then listed on a rank order question sheet in order to identify the issues of importance to both users and the student nurses; forty users and forty student nurses were contacted for the question sheets to be completed. Tables 5.4 to 5.9 show the result of that exercise. From Tables 5.5, 5.7 and 5.9 it can be seen more clearly what the top five ranked issues are, firstly from the users' and secondly the nurses' responses.

These results from the Rank Order Exercise are presented in order to focus in on the key concerns and priorities that users and nurses have identified for practice if real partnership working is to prevail. The intent has been to provide the real voice of the service users and not one of practitioners' views of the needs of users. The views of users are contrasted with the views of nurses who are on the front line of service delivery, to ascertain the degree of convergence or divergence between the different parties. At the heart of the 1994 Review of Mental Health

Table 5.4 Comparative figures with respect to what nurses should 'do'

	Users N (%)	Nurses N (%)
Promote activities/group work	14 (35)	5 (12.5)
Listen to users as individuals	25 (62.5)	36 (90)
Boost confidence and independence	18 (45)	27 (67.5)
Improve user/nurse ratio	3 (7.5)	8 (20)
Give information	15 (37.5)	14 (35)
Spend more time with users	17 (42.5)	23 (57.8)
Develop a support network	9 (22.5)	18 (45)
Promote a positive image of mental illness	15 (37.5)	12 (30)
Engage in social skills training	6 (15)	3 (7.5)
Promote structure and safety	8 (20)	11 (27.5)
Manage aggression and show understanding	16 (40)	3 (7.5)
Offer counselling	11 (27.5)	12 (30)
Give medication	10 (25)	7 (17.5)
Show respect	22 (55)	21 (52.5)
Help with personal hygiene	11 (27.5)	0 (0)

Table 5.5 Top five ranked issues of importance with respect to what nurses 'do'

Do?	Users' views N (%)
1. Listen to users as individuals	25 (62.5)
2. Show respect	22 (55)
3. Boost confidence and independence	18 (45)
4. Spend more time with users	17 (42.5)
5. Manage aggression and show understanding	15 (40)

Do?	Nurses views N (%)
1. Listen to users as individuals	36 (90)
2. Boost confidence and independence	27 (67.5)
3. Spend more time with users	23 (57.5)
4. Show respect	21 (52.5)
5. Develop a support network	18 (45)

Table 5.6 Comparative figures regarding what nurses should 'be'

	Users N	(%)	Nurses N	(%)
Self aware and mature	23	(57.5)	32	(80)
Better educated	10	(25)	9	(22.5)
Sensitive and approachable	25	(26.5)	32	(80)
Advocate and change agent	3	(7.5)	25	(62.5)
Friendly and 'human'	28	(70)	13	(32.5)
Empathetic person first then a nurse	17	(42.5)	18	(45)
A specialist	10	(25)	4	(10)
Competent independent practitioner	5	(12.5)	20	(50)
More powerful/of greater influence	7	(17.5)	1	(2.5)
Paid more	10	(25)	8	(20)
Assertive	4	(10)	8	(20)
Available	19	(47.5)	15	(37.5)
Non threatening	20	(50)	9	(22.5)

Table 5.7 Top five ranked issues of importance regarding what nurses should 'be'

Be?	Users' views	
	N	(%)
1. Friendly and 'human'	28	(70.5)
2. Sensitive and approachable	25	(62.5)
3. Self aware and mature	23	(57.5)
4. Non threatening	20	(50)
5. Available	19	(47.5)
5. Interested in nursing as a career	19	(47.5)

Be?	Nurses' views	
	N	(%)
1. Self aware and mature	32	(80)
2. Sensitive and approachable	32	(80)
3. Advocate and change agent	25	(62.5)
4. Empathetic person first then a nurse	18	(45)
5. Available	15	(37.5)

Table 5.8 Comparative figures regarding what nurses should 'know'

	Users		Nurses	
	N	(%)	N	(%)
More about medical and physical problems	30	(75)	10	(25)
Communication skills	25	(62.5)	33	(82.5)
Themselves	10	(25)	30	(75)
Talking therapies	22	(55)	13	(32.5)
Counselling skills	15	(37.5)	21	(52.5)
Medication and its effects	26	(65)	26	(65)
Theory and research	7	(17.5)	18	(45)
Problem solving approaches	20	(50)	28	(70)
About different life experiences	26	(650)	18	(45)
Aspects of social work and occupational therapy	19	(47.5)	3	(7.5)

Table 5.9 Top five ranked issues of importance regarding what nurses should 'know'

Know?	Users' views	
	N	(%)
1. More about medical and physical problems	30	(75)
2. Medication and its effects	26	(65)
2. About different life experiences	26	(65)
3. Communication skills	25	(62.5)
4. Counselling skills	22	(55)
5. Problem solving approaches	20	(50)

Know?	Nurses' views	
	N	(%)
1. Communication skills	33	(82.5)
2. Themselves	30	(75)
3. Problem solving approaches	28	(70)
4. Medication and its effects	26	(65)
5. Counselling skills	21	(52.5)

Nursing *Working in Partnership: a collaborative approach to care* is the belief that 'Mental health nursing should re-examine every aspect of its policy and practice in the light of the needs of people who use the services' (Department of Health 1994 p48). The success of that policy in practice depends on first correctly identifying those needs.

These findings from the first stage of the research were then used in devising questionnaires for targeting a larger sample in the second stage, which is presented in the next chapter.

References

Allport G 1942 The use of personal documents in psychological science. Social Science Research Council, New York

Altschul A 1997 A personal view of psychiatric nursing. In: Tilley S (ed) The mental health nurse. Blackwell, London

Basch C E 1987 Focus group interview: an underutilised research technique for improving theory and practice in health education. Health Education Quarterly 14(4):411-448

Burnard P 1991 A method of analysing interview transcripts in qualitative research. Nurse Education Today 11:461-466

Department of Health 1994 Working in partnership - report of the Mental Health Nursing Review Team. HMSO, London

Edwards K 1999 A study of pre-registration nursing students and users of mental health services. (Unpublished PhD thesis). University of Birmingham

Epstein M, Olsen A 1999 An introduction to consumer politics. In: Clinton A, Nelson S (eds) Advanced practice in mental health nursing. Blackwell, London

Feldman M S 1995 Strategies for interpreting qualitative data. Sage, Thousand Oaks

Folch-Lyon E, Trost J 1981 Conducting focus group sessions. Student Family Planning Part 1 12:443-449

Glaser B, Strauss A L 1967 The discovery of grounded theory. Aldine, New York

Glaser B, Strauss A L 1968 The discovery of grounded theory: strategies for qualitative research. Widenfeld and Nicolson, London

Jick T D 1993 Mixing qualitative and quantitative: triangulation in action. In: Van Maanen L (ed) Qualitative methodology. Sage, London

Lincoln Y S, Guba E G 1985 Naturalist enquiry. Sage, California

Morse L M 1994 Emerging from the data: the cognitive processes of analysis in qualitative enquiry. In: Morse J M (ed) Critical issues in qualitative research methods. Sage, London

Nolan P 1993 A history of mental health nursing. Chapman and Hall, London

Nyswander D B 1982 Group dynamics, health education monographs no.19. In: Simonds S K (ed) SOPHE heritage collection of health education monographs, the philosophical, behavioural and professional basis for health education. Oakland, California, ch 1

Oppenheim A M 1992 Questionnaire design, interviewing and attitude measurement. Pinter, London

Osgood C E, Tannenbaum P H 1955 The principle of congruity in the prediction of attitude change. Psychological Review 62:42-55

Powers B A, Knapp T R 1990 A dictinary of nursing theory and research. Sage, London

Rogers A, Pilgrim D 1994 Service users views of psychiatric nurses. British Journal of Nursing 3(1):16-18

Stevens P J M, Schade A L, Chalk B, Slevin O D A 1993 Understanding research. Campion, Edinburgh

Taylor S, Bogdan R 1984 Introduction to qualitative research methods: the search for meaning, 2nd edn. Wiley, New York

Turner B 1981 Some practical aspects of qualitative data analysis: one way of organising the cognitive processes associated with the generation of grounded theory. Quality and Quantity 15:222-247

White E 1990 The future of psychiatric nursing by the year 2000: a Delphi study. Department of Nursing, University of Manchester

Chapter 6

What should a mental health nurse do, be and know?

INTRODUCTION

The second phase of this research was the collecting of data by way of questionnaires constructed from the information collected and presented in the previous chapter. Again, the process of data collection is described so that the means of arriving at a conclusion is made transparent to the reader. Following on from the information gleaned via the focus group interviews and the rank order exercise it was decided to construct questionnaires from that information for the purpose of targeting a larger group, thus combining both qualitative and quantitative research techniques. A total of 200 service users and 200 students of nursing studies were targeted and participated in the research. It was considered essential to construct the questionnaires from the first phase of the data collecting process so that they reflected the issues that the participants wanted on the agenda in relation to the research questions and so that that agenda would be taken forward as areas for further research. An existing standardised questionnaire designed for other purposes was, therefore, deemed inappropriate. Also a preordained questionnaire may not have been sensitive to the current climate in which user sensitivity, working in partnership and user centredness is high on the health and social care agenda. The need for research to reflect a user perspective has been commented upon in reports such as *Caring for People* (Department of Health 1989), *The Health of the Nation* (Department of Health 1991) and *Working in Partnership* (Department of Health 1994) as well as MIND's and other user groups' initiatives that have been concerned about the empowerment of those that use mental health services and to ensure that such services are responsive to their expressed needs. In order to achieve empowerment as a health care goal it is necessary to understand the perspective of the target group. Theorising about empowerment and partnership is one thing, making it a reality is quite another.

The design of the questionnaire followed the themes of the Focus Groups, 'what should a nurse do, be and know', as well as incorporating questions that sought to obtain biographical information. All types of questions have advantages and disadvantages. Open questions can contain more complete answers, but can be difficult to answer and analyse. Closed questions can be easier to answer and analyse but may not contain the full range of possible answers. In consideration of this a Likert scale was employed in offering the respondents the opportunity to indicate their attitude towards particular statements by choosing one of a small number of ordered alternatives. At the end of each section of the questionnaire there was an open-ended statement that invited the respondents to make any other comment that they would like to make.

PILOT STUDY

Piloting is essential to all research in that it gives the researcher the opportunity to practise and evaluate the proposed data collecting instruments and make other necessary changes revealed by the pilot study. As the questionnaires were designed using the data collected through the Focus Groups, they had not been validated or had their reliability tested. Therefore, the pilot study was undertaken in order to establish the validity and reliability of the instruments. The research aimed to target a total number of 200 users and 200 students as according to McIver (1991) 'as a rule, the more variation in the people who are to be given the questionnaire, the greater the sample size needs to be so that there are enough people in each category to make comparison possible'. She suggests that the larger the sample size, the less the error and the rate of error decrease slows down around the 400 mark. For the purpose of this research, due to the time constraint and the small numbers that made up many of the user groups, it was decided to target a total population of 400 made up of 200 users and 200 students. The piloting of the questionnaires initially obtained a 10% sample of both target groups.

Nursing students were approached by contacting Colleges and Universities in a random manner working from Applicant Handbooks and again opportunism influenced the selection process with those that responded earliest being pursued and engaged with. The researcher travelled to the various locations to meet with the groups and asked them to complete the questionnaires. Communication had already taken place with the responsible tutor for the particular group and the time and a venue had been arranged in advance at the particular institution. Therefore, it was relatively uncomplicated to obtain responses as there was a captive audience which was prepared to co-operate. No major methodological problems ensued. As a result of the pilot study, slight changes had to be made to the questionnaire. Some questions were perceived as ambiguous and the layout also needed modifying. Once the changes had been made another group was contacted which comprised 18 nursing students who were asked to complete the questionnaire and after further adjustments the questionnaire was used as the instrument for the main target group of 200 students.

The same principle of random and opportunistic sampling from the lists of user groups were applied to engaging with users, although it was much more difficult and time consuming to gain access as they were not a captive audience in the sense that the nursing students were. Again a 10% sample was targeted and the researcher quickly became aware that some users were experiencing difficulties with the wording of the questions as well as the layout and they made suggestions for a more user-friendly questionnaire. The researcher found that respondents posed rational questions and gave rational answers and users' state of mind did not appear to be a major problem as it is sometimes assumed when users' views are sought. That had also been found in a study by Raphael (1977).

After modification, another two user groups, totalling 21, were contacted from those that had already expressed an interest in participating and the responses revealed that the design of the questionnaire was now more user friendly. Further minor adjustments were made and the questionnaire was adopted for use with the main target groups.

Questionnaires

The words used in compiling the questions were primarily those which the groups had used during the first phase of data collection and as a result of piloting. There was concern within the groups as to how certain words could be operationalised; 'kind' and 'understanding' were two such words but some users made it quite clear that by 'kind' they meant compassionate, gentle and not being cruel. Some users felt that they had experienced cruelty when in hospital and that they should have been treated with much more sensitivity and consideration. Cruelty was mainly referred to in a psychological sense and kindness was a word that they felt described what they wanted. On the question relating to 'kindness' some respondents queried its validity and felt it was not specific enough or suggested that it was paternalistic. By the term 'understanding' users meant that nurses seldom took the time or effort to genuinely comprehend how users' mental health problems really affected them as individuals. Users felt that in the main they were only being understood as a diagnostic entity and that issue needed to be on the agenda. The importance of both words was acknowledged and despite the difficulties in operationalising such terms the groups felt that they should be included in the questionnaires to obtain information about how respondents may interpret them.

Initially, it proved difficult to get the right balance between wording that might be considered too elementary and patronising and wording that might appear too academic and jargonistic. Some users felt that the words and questions were over simplified because they were stereotyped as 'ex-psychiatric patients' with little insight or intellect. They suggested that it was not necessary to use a simplified language, although, conversely, some users felt that the wording of the questionnaires was not their language and it needed simplifying for them to understand what was being asked. Methodologically, this was difficult to reconcile and one of the reasons why the researcher went with the questionnaires rather than sending them by post was to be available to clarify any issues that may have arisen or to clarify questions that seemed ambiguous when the questionnaires were being completed. The intention was to communicate as clearly and simply as possible so as to achieve an optimum response rate without wasting too much time or effort. As Burnard (1994) points out, 'we write to communicate and if we do not write clearly, we do not communicate. Instead we confuse'. One user offered the following advice in relation to the questionnaires: 'If you hope to get them returned you need to keep them short, straightforward and without any jargon and come along and meet with people so that they can ask any questions, as we are doing now, otherwise, they will be thrown in the corner over there with the rest of them'. A graveyard of questionnaires was clearly visible.

Targeting groups

In the targeting of user groups the process was largely opportunistic and influenced by Snowball sampling, since the groups that had been part of the first stage were quite free in offering other contact names and addresses. In the order in which responses were received arrangements were made to meet with the various groups although an attempt was made to ensure geographical diversity and differences between the groups. A low response rate is one of the biggest problems with questionnaire studies, especially when they are sent through the post. For example, the European Regional Council of the World Federation for Mental Health in 1996 reported that a group from Mind-Link UK used a questionnaire to survey all their 1,400 members and only 239 responded and of these only 107 were 80% complete, revealing the limitation of postal surveys. In endeavouring to avoid that problem in this research, the researcher arranged to meet with participants so that the questionnaires could be completed and returned immediately. A face-to-face approach does provide a better response rate but there are inherent dangers that one has to be cautious of. For example, subjects may respond in a way that they think the researcher wants them to respond. The researcher was careful not to be leading or directive while responding to questions or in clarifying issues that were raised.

Engaging with some of the user groups proved to be very time consuming in terms of phone calls, letter writing and waiting for responses. Users often questioned the motive for the research. At that time the researcher published an article about the first phase of the research and subsequently enclosed it with the letters of request to meet with other groups. That produced a noticeably swifter response and invitations to meet with the various groups as it served to clarify the researcher's position and agenda and engendered trust. From a data collection perspective this was welcomed but equally one became aware of reactivity and what has become known as the 'Hawthorn Effect' and the need to guard against it. Whilst meeting with the respondents, the researcher was careful not to influence the responses by expressing or disclosing a perspective on any of the issues. During the meetings much unsolicited, peripheral yet noteworthy material was mentioned that provided a rich source of data that would otherwise be lost if not recorded. Thus, field notes were vital and were also used to enhance understanding of pertinent issues that were not revealed by written responses to the questions.

Application handbooks were again used to identify and target student nurses in the latter part of their course, and opportunism influenced the selection process, since those who responded earliest were pursued and engaged with. A guiding principle had been to try and select institutions in a manner that gained a wide geographical spread. The questionnaires were administered to the student nurse groups in the same method as that employed for the user groups, except the assistance of some tutors was sought. They volunteered to administer the questionnaires to the groups for whom they were responsible. That reduced demands on travelling and made more time available to the researcher for engaging with service users, who unlike the student nurses were not a captive audience.

STAGE 2: FINDINGS

This section looks first at the actual data collecting process and at some of the data from the field notes that were recorded after the meetings for questionnaire completion. The findings will then be presented in a way that reflects the structure of the questionnaires, commencing with biographical details, followed by what a nurse should do, be and know. The response rate achieved was 100% with 400 questionnaires being completed, although there is some missing data as not all questions were answered.

Initial problems arose with the first user group that responded to the request to meet with them. The key person who had organised the meeting had been readmitted into hospital. Only three participants turned up for the planned meeting and two were very concerned about filling in any kind of form without the regular chairperson being there. They stated that they could only talk unofficially, thus sadly projecting feelings of dependency rather than of empowerment or working in partnership. The third person was more independent and completed the questionnaire. He felt that they should do things for themselves and work with the researcher. On returning to meet with this group ten service users were present and, as previously planned, they were all prepared to participate and completed the questionnaire.

Another group apologised for anything they said which caused offence, stressing that some nurses were very good. What they identified about the 'very good' nurses was that it was something to do with their individual attitudes and personalities and little to do with how services were organised. This was an issue that re-emerged with many of the groups. Another common and consistent theme was that users did not feel that nurses took their 'illness' and individual suffering seriously. They felt that nurses were quite content to function within the boundary of a medical model and diagnostic labels and belittled users' concerns as simply part of their pathology. Insufficient time spent with users whilst in hospital was another issue that was often mentioned in peripheral conversation by both users and nursing students. This was a concern that had been identified during the first stage of the research and highlighted as one of the five top ranked issues during the Rank Order Exercise. The need for human contact was expressed as an important matter and a number of users suggested that one of the benefits of participating with user groups was that it helped to establish a support network, as such groups offered support, information, and partnership and were often experienced as a surrogate extended family.

An Obsessive Compulsive Disorder Self-Help Group expressed opinions that, in their experience, nurses did not have sufficient specialist knowledge and, as a result, treated their disorder as if they could simply stop being obsessional if they so chose. They deliberated upon life experience, maturity and age and reached a consensus within the group that mental health students should preferably be over thirty. They considered that, at that age, nurses would be sufficiently mature to have gained some insight into the pressures of everyday life and an understanding of how some people may develop what can be regarded as inappropriate behaviour. Another group's (Consumer Action Group) primary concern was to do with the selection process of student nurses and the discontinuing of unsuitable candidates once they are on nursing courses. That group did not feel that there was any effective monitoring of the student nurse's development once they had secured a place on a course and that they would qualify regardless of their aptitude. Another group seemed very surprised, yet pleased, to see someone coming from quite a distance, on a cold wet evening to ask them for their opinions and were encouraged that someone may take their views seriously and influence the quality of services that they received. Therefore, they felt that they had a responsibility to complete the questionnaire and to be as open and honest as they possibly could. An 'Ex Patient' support group, (this was the name that they had chosen for themselves) primarily concerned with problems relating to alcohol and drug abuse, held a regular monthly meeting on hospital premises. Thirty-five users were in attendance. Their discussion reflected their concerns that there were moves afoot from the particular Health Care Trust to stop them using the premises. The group perceived that they were seen to be becoming too independent and powerful, making service demands and excluding professionals from their meetings. This latter point was not strictly true as professionals were invited to attend if it was felt that they needed to be there to contribute to a particular issue of concern. An alternative venue away from the hospital premises had been offered to the group but they felt that relocation would undermine the support group, as the current venue was easily accessible by public transport. The group suggested that it was important to communicate openly with anyone interested in their welfare, as they believed that it was vital to involve others who may be able to influence outcomes and improve the service. Other groups expressed similar feelings and concerns and overall the majority of participants felt that it was more in their interest to participate in research than not to, since only by speaking out could they hope to have any influence over any future development of mental health services. There were some users, however, who were dismissive of anyone doing research from a professional background and indicated a great deal of distrust in motives and outcomes.

Engaging with most of the nursing students for the completion of questionnaires was relatively structured and organised. Time had been set aside within their programme to meet with the researcher if they so wished. Therefore, less peripheral discussion took place with the students than had occurred with the users. Many students did express opinions about their preparation for their future role and felt that the educational input was of a better quality to that received by previous generations of nurses. Comments were also made about practice not being up to the standards suggested by their educational input.

Respondents' biographical details

The following biographical data is important in attempting to establish how representative the participants were and whether there were significant differences between users and students with respect to age, sex, marital status, living arrangements, ethnic origins, admissions and duration of admissions. The implication of that data is to determine whether or not details such as class, gender, age, race and marital status, which provide the context of user/nurse interactions, have a bearing on how users experience nursing staff. Horwitz (1983) suggests that the greater the personal differences between people the more likely they are to ascribe certain labels that have a devaluing and negative effect upon them. It has also been suggested by Strauss and Corbin (1988) and Handyside and Heyman (1994) that people with chronic mental health problems and professional carers tend to inhabit fundamentally dissimilar worlds, which may have implications for how professional care givers are able to respond to users in an understanding and non-judgemental manner.

Table 6.1 Age of respondents

Age range	Users	Nurses	Total
18–20	4 (2%)	7 (3.5)	11 (5.5%)
21–30	28 (14%)	118 (59%)	146 (73%)
31–40	56 (28%)	48 (24%)	104 (52%)
41–50	56 (28%)	26 (13%)	82 (41%)
51–60	36 (18%)	1 (0.5%)	37 (18.5%)
61–65	13 (6.5%)		13 (6.5%)
65+	7 (3.5%)		7 (3.5%)
Total Numbers	200	200	400

The above table gives a breakdown of the age of users and students. The majority of the students are in the age categories 21–30 (59%) and 31–40

(24%), whilst the majority of users are in the 31–40 (28%) and 41–50 (28%) groups. From these figures one can observe that the nursing sample in this study appears to be recruiting from a slightly older age group than the traditional 18–19-year-old candidates that made up the bulk of recruits in the past. There are only 3.5% (n=7) of students within the 18–20 categories while there are 13% (n=26) in the 41–50 group. These figures indicate that there is an overall increase in the age of those now entering nursing within this sample. In response to the question about the perceived ideal age of a nurse and its relevance, only 128 users stipulated a specific age but of those responses the mean age was calculated at 34.6 years. Only 111 nursing students identified a specific age in response to the same question, with the age being identified between 17 and 60+ years. From these only 7 suggested that under the age of 20 was a suitable age to train to be a mental health nurse. The mean was calculated to be 30.5 years as the desirable age. These figures have to be considered in the context of some of the written remarks that were made in response to questions that asked for any further comments, as demonstrated by the following quote:

'Depends on the person not their age; I do not think it matters, any age if they care and respect people as individuals; different people mature at different ages; life experience and approachability are more important than age; can you put an ideal age range on maturity?'

Table 6.2 Gender

	Users	Std Nurses	Total
Male	98 (49%)	63 (31.5%)	161
Female	98 (49%)	136 (68%)	234
*		1 (0.5%)	1
Total	**196 (98%)	200 (100%)	396

* One respondent answered 'other' in response to this question.
** Number of missing observations: 4.

Table 6.2 relating to gender, shows that there are equal numbers of male 49% (n=98) and female 49% (n=98) users who participated in this study. This was coincidental and not by design. The nursing students, as expected, were predominately female; 68% (n=136) female, 31.5% (n=63) male. Pilgrim and Rogers (1993) have suggested that more women are diagnosed as being mentally ill than men and Busfield (1996) asserts that women are frequently assumed to be more prone to mental disorder than men but intimates that evidence shows a much more complex gender landscape of mental disorder, with men and women manifesting different types of problems. There is much debate as to the reason for gender differences but that is beyond the scope of this book.

Table 6.3 Ethnic origins

	Users	Std Nurses	Total
African		6 (3%)	6
Afro–Caribbean	1 (0.5%)	6 (3%)	7
Asian	4 (2%)	5 (2.5%)	9
British	162 (81%)	160 (80%)	322
Irish	21 (10.5%)	15 (7.5%)	36
Other	12 (6%)	8 (4%)	20
Total	200 (100%)	200 (100%)	400

With respect to the ethnic origins of the participants, 81% (n=162) of users and 80% (n=160) of student nurses responded that they were British. Those from ethnic minorities were 19% (n=38) users and 20% (n=40) student nurses, although there was an absence of Africans and Afro-Caribbeans represented within the user groups.

Table 6.4 Marital status

	Users	Std Nurses	Total
Single	98 (49%)	99 (49.5%)	197
Married	40 (20%)	59 (29.5%)	99
Cohabiting	12 (6%)	21 (10.5%)	33
Separated	41 (20.5%)	18 (9%)	59
Widowed	8 (4%)	1 (0.5%)	9
Total	199 (99.5%)	198 (99%)	397

Table 6.4 shows that 197 of the total sample population are single with a relatively even distribution between users 49% (n=98) and students 49.5% (n=99). Of those that are either married or cohabiting 26% (n=52) are users and 40% (n=80) are nurses. The personal differences between the users' and the students' marital composition does not appear to be great but the difference in marital status between users and students must be considered in the context of age. The students are overall much younger than the users, therefore their single status may be more likely as they fall nearer the average age of marriage (Men 30.5 and women 28.2, Office for National Statistics, 2000) or it may be that for the students embarking on a new career it is their choice to be single. One cannot conclude that the students are sharing the life experiences of users because they are single. To be older and single has a certain social stigma and involves practical difficulties such as the reduced availability of social venues for the older age groups to meet. The fact that users are older and single may reflect difficulties for them in forming relationships. Some users suggested that the lack of opportunity to find a partner might be due to the stigma associated with having been diagnosed as suffering from a mental illness. One can see that more users than students have been separated, 20.5% (n=41) and 9% (n=18) respectively. As users were older this might be expected.

Table 6.5 Living arrangements

	Users	Std Nurses	Total
Alone	66 (33%)	58 (29%)	124
With children	9 (4.5%)	18 (9%)	27
Spouse/partner	49 (24.5%)	79 (39.5%)	128
Parents	24 (12%)	12 (6%)	36
Other*	52 (26%)	32 (16%)	84
Total	200 (100%)	199 (99.5%)	399

* Other: Group home, hostel, sheltered accommodation.

Table 6.5 shows that 33% (n=66) of users and 29% (n=58) of students live alone while others did have some form of company. Although the figures are relatively even, the number of users, 4.5% (n=9), who live with their children is half that of the students, 9% (n=18). The 'other' category for the user group is greater than for the students, 25.5% (n=51) and 16% (n=32) respectively. The Central Statistical Office (National Statistic Office 2003) specifies that there has been a pattern of increasing single households since the early 1960s and in the 2001 Census one-person households had increased to 30% (6.5 million) from 26.3% in 1991. Nearly half of the one-person households (3.1 million) are one-pensioner only households and three-quarters of these (2, 366,000) are occupied by a woman living on her own. However, in the remaining 3, 376, 000 one-person households, male occupants outnumber women by three to two. More than one in eight of single-person households do not have central heating – this amounts to over 383, 000 pensioners and over 430, 000 non-pensioners. Over 70, 000 single-person households do not have sole use of a bath/shower and toilet – 21, 000 of these being pensioners. More than half of pensioners living alone have a limiting long-term illness (52.8 per cent). Such social circumstances will inevitably affect people's mental and physical health and must be borne in mind when planning individuals' health care needs.

Tables 6.6 and 6.7 give the number of admissions to a psychiatric hospital and the duration of user involvement as an indication of the representativeness of the users' views in terms of their experience of the service. This data is important to illustrate that the opinions from this research represent a considerable amount of experience of mental health services and, as such, the views cannot simply be dismissed as ill informed.

Table 6.6 illustrates that in response to the question relating to a history of a mental illness only 20 students responded that they had been users of mental health services, and only 17 responded to the subsequent question relating to the duration of contact with the service. In one group of 16 students, 6 refused to partake in the research as they felt that the questions on whether they had been users of mental health services were too intrusive, despite reassurance of the confidential and the anonymous nature of the questionnaire. Perhaps this was to be expected considering the Allitt Inquiry (Department of Health 1994b) that urged employers not to recruit candidates for nursing posts if they showed any evidence of a 'major personality disorder'. Many of the

Table 6.6 Number of admissions

Admissions	Users	Std nurses	Total
1	29 (15%)	4 (2%)	33
2	37 (18.5%)	1 (0.5%)	38
3	24 (12%)	0	24
4	32 (16%)	1 (0.5%)	33
5	12 (6%)	0	12
Other	59 (29.5)	13 (6.5%)	72
*		1 (0.5%)	1
Total	193	20 (10%)	213

Number of Missing Observations: 187
* One student acknowledged that she had been a user but did not select a category regarding the number of admissions.

nurses were conversant with the Beverly Allitt case and did not feel that being too honest was in their best interest. It is therefore understandable within such a climate that still prevails, for nurses to feel vulnerable in terms of gaining employment, their career opportunities and the possible discrimination and stigma against someone who has been a user of mental health services.

Table 6.7 suggests that student nurses' involvement with mental health services is limited in terms of time spent as recipients of such services.

From the initial agenda setting stage, service users had put forward the notion that those who had recovered from a mental health problem were probably more able to empathise and meet the needs of other service users if they were given the opportunity to become employed as part of the service providing team. Unfortunately, in the discussions and written comments many felt that a history of mental illness would result in them not being considered or entrusted with responsibility for the health of others and therefore, they would be excluded from pursuing a career in nursing. It may be that a greater number of students had been the recipients of mental health services than indicated by the above figures because of the concern about disclosing the fact. It is not known to what extent applicants to nursing with a history of mental illness are

Table 6.7 Duration of admissions

	Users	Std Nurses	Total
Less than 6 weeks	12	8	20
7 –12 weeks	15	4	19
13 –25 weeks	12	3	15
26–51 weeks	11	0	11
More than 52 weeks	147	1	148
*		1	1

Number of Missing Observations: 186
* One student responded without disclosing duration.

being screened via interviews and selection criteria, and thereby prevented from entering nursing, or whether information about a history of mental illness is not mentioned or ignored. However, there has been some positive movement regarding that issue since the Allitt Inquiry with an account in the *Nursing Times* (April 16, 1997) that a Mental Health Trust was 'actively seeking to recruit nurses who have experienced mental health problems as part of a ground-breaking initiative aimed at boosting equal opportunities for people with mental health problems'. They aimed for one in ten employees to be users or ex-users of mental health services. Subsequently, there was a backlash to that initiative with a spokesperson from the now defunct UKCC declaring that 'Practitioners with a history of mental ill health can be just as dangerous to patients as someone found guilty of serious professional misconduct' (Editorial 1997). The likely effect of that kind of response is to drive nurses with a history of mental health problems further into secretiveness and insecurity. One cannot stop nurses from having mental health problems, but one can stop them from being open and honest about those problems when their livelihood is at stake.

The minimum qualification for entering a nursing diploma course at present is 5 GCSEs or their equivalent. With the move towards degree level as the base qualification for nursing, in line with other graduate level courses the entry requirement is a minimum of 2 'A' levels. The pursuit of degree status as the base line currency in nursing has rapidly gathered momentum as has the promotion of education beyond registration and a move towards the concept of life-long learning. The intention is to produce reflective and questioning practitioners who may have more confidence and feel able to voice their views more articulately. Education is not just about knowledge per se but brings with it the confidence to question, challenge and influence the decision making processes, thus equipping nurses to act as agents for change to bring about a more effectively focused, user-centred service. Questions on academic achievement were initially included in both questionnaires, for users and nurses, but eventually excluded as a result of piloting since a majority of users felt that they would be 'shown up to be stupid' by their lack of qualifications.

User employment

The findings from this study show that of the 200 user respondents, 79.5% (n=159) were not engaged in any kind of employment, only 8.5% (n=17) were in full time work while 9% (n=18) were employed part time and the remaining 3% (n=6) were in rehabilitative sheltered work. This differed from the situation of the student nurses who had very good prospects of being employed on completion of their courses especially given the current shortage of mental health nurses. The employment status of any individual, whether or not they have experienced a significant mental health problem, is vital for people to feel a sense of integration and inclusion into mainstream society. Unfortunately, little interest is paid to employment issues when planning care, be it stress at work or opportunities of gaining work following a mental health problem.

The sections of the questionnaires relating to what a nurse should do, be and know were rated on a five point Likert scale.

FINDINGS ABOUT WHAT NURSES DO

Table 6.8 Distribution of answers (Users), 1 to indicate of little importance/helpfulness/disagree, 5 as very important/helpful/agree

Do	1 n (%)	2 n (%)	3 n (%)	4 n (%)	5 n (%)
1. How important is it to receive information regarding your treatment and care plan?	13(7.5)	6(3)	9(4.5)	24(12)	144(72)
2. From your experience how helpful have nurses been in supplying such information?	22(11)	39(19.5)	58(29)	17(8.5)	36(18)
3. How would you rate nurses' ability in running therapeutic groups?	25(12.5)	33(16.5)	66(33)	30(15)	29(14.5)
4. There may be times when a nurse has to physically restrain a service user, how do you value this role?	31(15.5)	27(13.5)	48(24)	32(16)	42(21)
5. How important is it for nurses to be educated/trained in counselling skills?	10(5)	1(0.5)	14(7)	19(9.5)	148(74)
6. How would you rate the role of the nurse in managing aggression?	20(10)	23(11.5)	58(29)	51(25.5)	59(29.5)
7. How important is it for nurses to spend planned time with users?	6(3)	4(2)	17(8.5)	27(13.5)	138(69)
8. How effective are nurses in dispelling a negative image of mental illness?	26(13)	25(12.5)	61(30.5)	30(15)	41(20.5)
9. How would you rate nurses in treating you as an individual?	26(13)	26(13)	63(31.5)	27(13.5)	43(21.5)
10. Nurses are always prepared to listen to you as a service user.	29(14.5)	58(29)	47(23.5)	29(14.5)	28(14)
11. How effective are nurses in motivating users?	27(13.5)	43(21.5)	59(29.5)	29(14.5)	17(8.5)
12. How helpful are nurses in involving family and/or significant others in your care?	47(13.5)	41(20.5)	46(23)	23(11.5)	31(15.5)
13. How important is it for family and/or significant others to be involved in your care?	12(6)	13(6.5)	30(15)	26(12)	106(53)
14. From your experience of psychiatric services how satisfactory was the user/nurse ratio?	29(14.5)	37(18.5)	55(27)	28(14)	34(17)

Table 6.9 Distribution of answers (Std/Nurses), 1 to indicate of little importance/ helpfulness/disagree, 5 as very important/helpful/agree

Do	1 n (%)	2 n (%)	3 n (%)	4 n (%)	5 n (%)

1. How would you rate nurses' ability in confidence building and promotion of independence for psychiatric patients/users?

    2(1)   9(4.5)   27(13.5)   44(22)   118(59)

2. How important are group activities for users?

    4(2)   16(8)   70(35)   110(55)

3. How important is 'kindness' towards users/patients?

    2(1)   1(0.5)   47(23.5)   51(25.5)   86(43)

4. How do you rate nurses' ability in treating users as individuals?

    4(2)   27(13.5)   89(44.5)   48(24)   28(14)

5. Should nurses spend more planned time talking with users?

    1(0.5)   3(1.5)   5(2.5)   44(22)   147(73.5)

6. The nurse/user ratio in hospital is satisfactory.

    7(3.5)   16(8)   38(19)   54(27)   84(42)

7. Social skills training is an essential role of the nurse.

    15(7.5)   21(10.5)   35(17.5)   50(25)   76(38)

8. Nurses are always prepared to listen to the views of service users.

    2(1)   0(0)   2(1)   50(25)   146(73)

9. Are nurses effective in dispelling a negative image of mental illness?

    3(1.5)   53(26.5)   110(55)   30(15)   4(2)

10. How important is the physical environment for care giving?

    1(0.5)   1(0.5)   16(8)   82(41)   100(50)

11. Is it important to involve family and/or significant others in the care process?

    0(0)   0(0)   13(6.5)   55(27.5)   132(66)

12. User/patient personal hygiene is a key role of the nurse.

    18(9)   39(19.5)   80(40)   45(22.5)   16(8)

13. Should users be given full information regarding treatment and care plan?

    12(6)   15(7.5)   16(8)   35(17.5)   122(61)

Throughout this research, the topic of information, or more precisely the lack of information, was alluded to by users who during various discussions felt that to be better informed would enable them to take greater control over their own lives and enter into realistic partnership working. Hence, in response to the question on the importance of information with respect to care planning and treatment, 72% (144) of the users stated that they considered this to be very important. However, in response to the subsequent question as to the helpfulness of nurses in supplying such information, the results shown in Table 6.8(2) give a clear picture of users' experiences as recipients of information from nurses.

In rating nurses' ability in running therapeutic groups the findings were unsubstantial with a wide and relatively even range of responses from the users, shown in Table 6.8(3). Comments made in response to the type of therapeutic groups seen as being most beneficial were:

- Groups that focused upon day-to-day problems, for example accommodation issues and how they can occupy their days in a worthwhile manner rather than in mundane irrelevant activities, which is what users often perceived/experienced within hospital settings.
- Social skills training, especially in relation to issues of gaining worthwhile employment, help with claiming benefits and leisure pursuits.

The student responses to the question on group activities, Table 6.9(2), veered to the very important category but their comments focused mainly upon activities such as art and crafts and, as one comment suggested, 'anything that stops them sitting around smoking all day'. The response to the question about whether social skills training is an essential role of the nurse elicited some confusion about whether this was part of the nurse's role or the role of the occupational therapist. Table 6.9(7) shows that the students' responses are skewed in support of the belief that social skills training is an essential role of the nurse. However, written comments expressed concern that if they had a claim to such a role then they really needed much more effective training in developing social skills training programmes themselves. Students were very positive with respect to the need for confidence building and the promotion of independence, which was rated highly, Table 6.9(1). The themes that the students identified in their written comments as to how these could be achieved were the following:

- A need to improve communication with users in an open and honest manner.
- Treat users more as individuals with individual needs and abilities and engage in meaningful activities.
- Involve significant others and maintain contact with users' localities.
- Be realistic and focused about housing, retraining and employment options.
- A need to refer to research and endeavour to apply relevant findings and to acknowledge the need for specialist-trained staff that are competent and confident.

In response to the question relating to physical restraint, there was a wide spread of responses, Table 6.8(4). Users did comment that there was a need for such interventions from time to time and that it could be experienced as something reassuring and protective. However, the manner in which it was generally done was of great concern and as one user commented, 'it is like being mugged by a gang in the street'.

A question that had been posed to the students was about the importance of 'kindness', Table 6.9(3). As mentioned, there had been problems trying to define that word but nevertheless it was included in the questionnaire. This word had arisen during the first phase of the research with much discussion within the user groups around doing things with 'kindness' as the following quote from a questionnaire illustrates, 'All I look for in a nurse is kindness and a willingness to help and to understand me. Although I have found some nurses to be open and caring, this needs to be the case all the time with all nurses.' The response to the question by the students was skewed towards the very important, but not in a convincing way, although this may be due to the nature of the question. There were many comments made that ranged from not really knowing what was being implied by 'kindness' to others expressing a need for it to be at the forefront of caring.

Table 6.8(5) shows that counselling was considered very important by 74% (n=148) of users and that they thought nurses should be educated and trained in counselling skills. Sixty-nine per cent (n=138) of users also responded that it was very important for nurses to spend 'planned time' with them and not to respond with a 'I'm really too busy approach', Table 6.8(7). Many of the users' comments suggested that nurses did respond in that way. The students' response to the idea of spending more 'planned time' talking with users was positive with 73.5% (n=147) regarding it as very important, Table 6.9(5). There were also many comments made by the students that referred to the lack of time, especially planned time, that was available to spend with users due to the pressure of administrative work.

Within the written comments by users, concern was expressed about the effectiveness of nurses in dispelling the negative image and the stigma of mental illness, Table 6.8(8). The general themes that emerged from users about that issue were the following:

- A need to be aware of unfolding current developments, user focused care and to endeavour to influence its progress.
- Get to know users as people with problems that need addressing, not cases that can or can not be cured, and disregard stereotypes of mental illness.
- Share information to enhance understanding of both users and carers, with the latter being much more involved.
- Listen to users and hear what they really have to say.

The student nurses shared the users' views in acknowledging the importance of making progress to dispel the negative image of mental illness, Table 6.9(9). They commented on the undesirable labelling of users as 'schizophrenics' or 'psychopaths'. The students also acknowledged that there was a real need for change. This conclusion led from their clinical experiences, their reading of current literature and the educational culture to which they were being exposed.

The question relating to nurses 'treating users as individuals' showed a wide distribution of results from both users and students, suggesting a lack of consistency and understanding on this issue, Tables 6.8(9) and 6.9(4). There were only two written comments provided by the students: 'Not seen much of that during my placements' and 'vast variations'.

Users suggested that they experienced being responded to mainly in a standardised 'production line' and frequently unhelpful manner. The response to the question regarding the importance of listening skills also showed that there was divergence on this issue between how users and the student nurses rate the preparedness of nurses to listen, Tables 6.8(10) and 6.9(8). The response from users indicates that they tended not to agree that nurses were prepared to listen, especially when they were experiencing disturbances and distress. This was their experience of practice. The students strongly agreed that nurses were prepared to listen but this may reflect the theory taught and what they believe nurses should do rather than what actually happens in practice. Two quotes by users may also throw some light on the issue and, in particular, reflect that the value for users in being listened to is that nurses then act on what they have to say:

> 'Shortly after entering hospital I was advised by my doctor to return to work and receive a regular injection and a visit from a nurse. For the following years I endured torture at work and not once did my CPN advise me about any benefits that I could claim if I went off sick. All he told me to do was to pull my socks up, I don't think he ever listened to me and I will never forgive him for that.'

> 'I had a good rapport with my nurse and this has probably helped to establish contact with my family. He is like a friend, he listens to me and he is flexible. He helped me sort out my debts and he gets things done. I am very grateful.'

Comments from the students help to elucidate their perspective on the issue of listening:

> 'I feel that if there are more nurses then they would feel more willing to use their skills. Nurses also need more support but no one listens to us.'

> 'It is only by listening that you will know what their needs are.'

The helpfulness of nurses in involving family and/or significant others in care had an inverse relationship with users' response to the question of the importance for family and/or significant others to be involved in care, Tables 6.8(12) and 6.9(11). Users responses were skewed towards the unhelpful in relation to nurses involving families while in relation to the latter question they veer towards wanting significant others to be involved, Table 6.8(13). This suggests a need that is unmet and at the heart of partnership working. However, users did not rate the importance of involving others as highly as the students, who saw this as an important part of maintaining a support network. There was much divergence on this issue and from the biographical details it can be seen that some users did not have any family to involve.

During this research the participants had regularly spoken about the question of whether there was a satisfactory nurse/user ratio in the provision of care. However, the findings show that there was much uncertainty about that issue with a wide spread of responses from both groups of participants, Tables 6.8(14) and 6.9(6). Although the student nurses indicated that it was of concern, their responses were not as conclusive as they could have been. The students felt that the current situation made too many administrative demands upon their time. Many of the comments from users and students indicated that increasing the nurse–user ratio would not really address the issue. One user had the following to say on this matter: 'the ratio of nurses is an insignificant point unless the nursing is effective with them listening to your expressed needs and being able to respond'. Interestingly, some of the comments from the students not only supported this position but also suggested that 'In general there are adequate staffing levels, but time needs to be managed appropriately, there is not always a need for more nurses but rather a change in ward and unit policy, a different skill mix, better trained, motivated and aware staff who are more client than doctor orientated, a need for more "good" nurses not "bad" ones who are there to engage with the users'.

A thematic analysis was applied to the final question in the section regarding what nurses do: 'If there is anything else that you would like to add to this section, please use the space below'. Issues were identified and integrated into general themes. Some issues appeared to be more distinct than others. The following is a presentation of that information in ranked order, in terms of the number of times the topics were mentioned, that reflects both users' and nursing students' views:

1. Greater involvement with users and their carers on all aspects of care.
2. Individual's attitudes need to be open and honest.
3. Too much administration and paperwork.
4. Less emphasis on medication but clearer and concise explanation of its purpose when it is used.

This section of the questionnaire endeavoured to ascertain the importance of certain characteristics for a mental health nurse and the following tables show the responses to the questions.

FINDINGS ABOUT WHAT NURSES SHOULD 'BE'

Be	1 n (%)	2 n (%)	3 n (%)	4 n (%)	5 n (%)
1. Self aware	6(3)	7(3.5)	37(18.5)	40(20)	99(49.5)
2. Older	39(19.5)	26(13)	54(27)	26(12)	39(19.5)
3. Knowlegeable	11(5.5)	6(3)	43(21.5)	45(22.5)	82(41)
4. Approachable	5(2.5)	3(1.5)	14(7)	25(12.5)	142(71)
5. Specialist	9(4.5)	14(7)	28(14)	43(21.5)	99(49.5)

Table 6.10 Distribution of answers (Users), 1 to indicate of little importance/ helpfulness/disagree, 5 as very important/helpful/agree

6. More individual authority to make decisions

| | 16(8) | 18(9) | 63(31.5) | 39(19.5) | 54(27) |

7. Change agent	13(6.5)	14(7)	48(24)	50(25)	60(30)
8. Assertive	10(5)	11(5.5)	39(19.5)	64(32)	57(28.5)
9. Sensitive	1(0.5)	3(1.5)	15(7.5)	34(17)	136(68)
10.Better paid	10(5)	1(0.5)	31(15.5)	44(22)	98(49)

Table 6.11 Distribution of answers (Std/Nurses), 1 to indicate of little importance/helpfulness/disagree, 5 as very important/helpful/agree

Be	1 n (%)	2 n (%)	3 n (%)	4 n (%)	5 n (%)
1. Approachable	2(1)	1(0.5)	0(0)	21(10.5)	176(88)
2. In nursing as a career not just a job	1(0.5)	1(0.5)	27(13.5)	85(42.5)	84(42)
3. Older	35(17.5)	29(14.5)	70(35)	36(18)	14(7)
4. Self aware	4(2)	2(1)	4(2)	44(22)	144(72)
5. Compassionate	10(5)	1(0.5)	31(15.5)	44(22)	98(49)
6. Specialist	3(1.5)	2(1)	37(18.5)	76(38)	78(39)
7. Advocate	4(2)	4(2)	21(10.5)	60(30)	111(55.5)
8. Understanding	2(1)	1(0.5)	5(2.5)	56(28)	135(67.5)

The first question for users related to self-awareness with 69.5% (n=139) indicating that they felt it was either an important or a very important variable in the preparation of nurses, Table 6.10(1). This compares with 94% (n−188) of the students' responses, Table 6.11(4). Comments made by two students were:

'I see it as important to know myself and to be aware of myself. I find it difficult to concede the possibility of knowing another person if I do not first know myself. In order to develop empathy, self-knowledge is important. This course has taught me the skills of communication that I have come to believe to be the most important element of psychiatric nursing.'

'Nurses must be self aware as this provides the strength that is needed when dealing with mentally ill people. A nurse without this awareness may be unable to cope with some situations and be of no use to clients.'

Being approachable was the highest rated concern by both users and students in relation to what a nurse should 'be', Tables 6.10(4) and

6.11(1). Some verbatim statements may help to make that issue more explicit:

> 'I found some nurses to be very hard and uncaring when you approached them. However, student nurses and auxiliary staff tend to be more sensitive and compassionate towards patients.'

> 'Treat us with respect when we approach them, people are in emotional crisis and do not need condescending little Hitlers who really show no interest at crisis time.'

A comment by one student stated that:

> 'The nurse in charge on ward X was really nice and kind to the patients, but when she was not there some of the staff were rude and I would keep well away from them'.

Table 6.11(3) shows the findings in relation to users' responses to nurses being knowledgeable. Their written responses can be summarised into three clear themes. The first one referred to the need for nurses to have a thorough grasp of the whole ambit of classified mental disorders. This was often mentioned in the context of reflecting either individual diagnosis and/or concerns and interests regarding medical diagnosis and not understanding the diagnostic label that users had often been given. Users felt that nurses should be able to clarify what the label actually meant and be able to provide the information they wanted about how their problem had been defined. The second issue referred to the need for effective interpersonal skills to enhance working relationships and to facilitate information giving and understanding. Thirdly, comments supported the need for the underpinning of any treatment interventions by research findings rather than what was perceived as trial and error, or in the words of one user 'a hit and miss approach'. However, some users did express an appreciation for a 'play it by ear' approach, in that flexibility is important in applying a particular theory or intervention, there was recognition of the danger that practice may be based on myth and tradition rather than on reliable research findings.

The questions posed to users on the importance of assertiveness for nurses and the role of nurses as agents of change elicited indecisive results yet skewed towards the very important category, Table 6.10(7, 8). These issues were spoken about in the context of having the confidence to express opinions and not to feel disempowered but there were also negative concerns expressed by users about nurses being more assertive if it meant nurses exerting more power over them. For example one user suggested that 'Nurses can come across as jailers, they need to focus on the positive rather than thinking you are always aggressive'. A comment by a student nurse suggested that 'Acute services appear to be over concerned with medicating individuals and returning them to the community without improving their life skills or the context of their lives. Nurses must become more assertive and influential and help provide other therapies'.

The response set out in Table 6.10(9) shows that the need for sensitivity was highly rated by users. Sensitivity was an issue that users felt passionately about because it was not perceived as a regular attribute within practice and they expressed the need for it to be put on the agenda and given a much higher profile. Compassion was also a word that had been used frequently by users both during the first phase of the research and during the piloting stage. They emphasised that it was an important word to include in the questionnaire despite it being difficult to operationalise. Users remarked that it should be used in the questionnaires in the hope that nurses would stop and think about its meaning and hopefully internalise the concept and use it in their practice. Users considered compassion as a basic human quality that was often missing from their care from nurses and other health care professionals, which might suggest that some professionals do not want to, or are unable to get close to people in their care. Table 6.11(5) shows the responses to the question on the importance of compassion from the student nurses. Some of the comments written by the student nurses suggested that 'compassion is more important than any specialist knowledge' but that compassion is not always shown to patients, and another student expressed the following concern: 'It depends what you mean by compassionate, if you mean caring for patients then I agree but you must not get too involved with them'.

With regard to whether nurses should be better financially rewarded, users responded without doubt affirmatively but many comments were also made relating to value for money, Table 6.10(10). That issue had arisen on a number of occasions whilst meeting with the different groups of both users and students. The issue of concern and debate was whether a higher salary would result in attracting and retaining within nursing a higher calibre of nurse. It was expressed that, with the best intention in mind, money is nonetheless an important factor in whether one is attracted to nursing and equally whether one would want to remain within the occupation as a life-long career. A higher salary is only one variable but students did comment that it was an important one in determining their continued commitment. Some of the written comments suggested that it would be the most proficient nurses that would leave because of low salary since they would probably be much more marketable in other occupations. Some users commented that many nurses did not seem interested in the individuals for whom they cared, and that nursing was merely a job and 'a way of getting money'. The students had discussed that issue during the focus groups with much enthusiasm, although in terms of responding to the question on the questionnaire, the results were positively skewed but only one comment was written down by the students. The quote was: 'nurses should be paid more money according to a skilled performance'. There was no attempt to identify the criteria as to what was meant by a 'skilled performance'.

Other comments made at the end of this section regarding what a nurse should be can be summarised into the following three concerns:

1. Both users and students felt that there is a need for nurses to be better

listeners and to act upon expressed concerns. Empowerment, understanding and the need to empathise with the experience of being mentally ill were highlighted.

2. Nurses should give out information more freely and be more involved with users and represent them. The following quote illustrates that point; 'as a hazard of their job, nurses have a lot to cope with, but they must not forget to put the patient first. Generally they are pleasant but appear under qualified and unwilling to get involved with patients'. It was reported that there was a conflict of interest, with nurses claiming to be user advocates but being expected to function within the policy guidelines of the service. Users' comments suggested that they felt that policies were not always in their best interest.

3. Nursing staff must be approachable and more responsible for their actions, develop professionally and optimise the use of their resources in a client-centred manner.

The following comment from one of the students serves to show the perceived difficulty of change and how powerful the status quo can be: 'The questionnaire is about how nurses in mental health should aim to be but often they are sucked into the system and it takes a strong personality to maintain this sort of integrity'.

As previously mentioned, as a result of the qualitative data collection, of the three sections regarding what a nurse should do, be and know, it was the 'knowing' that received the least amount of attention and as a result there were fewer questions posed.

FINDINGS ABOUT WHAT NURSES SHOULD 'KNOW'

Table 6.12 Distribution of answers (Users), 1 to indicate of little importance/ helpfulness/disagree, 5 as very important/helpful/agree

Know	1 n (%)	2 n (%)	3 n (%)	4 n (%)	5 n (%)
1 Theory	10(5)	9(4.5)	39(19.5)	49(24.5)	79(39.5)
2. Research	8(4)	11(5.5)	46(23)	62(31)	61(30.5)
3. Knowledge of physical illnesses	11(5.5)	7(3.5)	21(10.5)	37(18.5)	116(58)
4. Awareness of social needs	3(1.5)	1(0.5)	15(7.5)	29(14.5)	141(70.5)
5. Occupational therapy activities	12(6)	6(3)	43(21.5)	43(21.5)	87(43.5)
6. Communication skills	4(2)	1(0.5)	13(6.5)	40(20)	134(67)
7. Problem solving skills	4(2)	2(1)	24(12)	57(28.5)	97(48.5)

8. Up-to-date with current issues

| | 6(3) | 7(3.5) | 32(16) | 48(24) | 91(45.5) |

9. Experience of life

| | 1(0.5) | 1(0.5) | 18(9) | 50(25) | 125(62.5) |

Table 6.13 Distribution of answers (Std/Nurses), 1 to indicate of little importance/helpfulness/disagree, 5 as very important/helpful/agree

Know	1 n (%)	2 n (%)	3 n (%)	4 n (%)	5 n (%)
1. Talking therapies	1(0.5)	2(1)	14(7)	87(43.5)	96(48)
2. Communication skills	1(0.5)	0(0)	1(0.5)	22(11)	176(88)
3. Knowledge of physical illnesses	8(4)	0(0)	49(24.5)	100(50)	43(22.5)
4. Counselling skills	0(0)	2(1)	9(4.5)	57(28.5)	132(66)
5. Medication	0(0)	4(2)	14(7)	62(31)	120(60)

The findings from the questionnaires have further confirmed that from a user perspective a specific professional psychiatric illness knowledge base is not high on their agenda. The weightiest response was to the question relating to awareness of social needs as shown at Table 6.12(4), which highlights the importance that users attach to the interpersonal rather than the intrapsychic domain.

Another notable finding that was rated highly by both users and student nurses with respect to what nurses should know related to communication skills, Tables 6.12(6) and 6.13(2). Users' comments indicated a concern that communications skills should be used within a structured therapeutic/counselling context and students' comments also reflected this view. One user comment suggested that,'Communication, counselling skills and self awareness are the foundations of a mental health nurse upon which anything else can be added'. The following written comments also illustrate users' concerns about communication and interpersonal relationships:

'I consider the nursing role of great importance, a person who is positive and calm and can communicate with friends and relatives is most important.'

'In my view the most important aspect of the suitability of an individual to be engaged as a psychiatric nurse lies in their aptitude and attitude to this kind of work. If an individual is unable to identify with the patients they should not be doing the job. The ability to relate to people, communicate and to listen and help them is something that cannot be taught, it may be possible to develop such skills but some people will never be able to learn them. Such people should not be employed as psychiatric nurses since you will never work with them in partnership but unfortunately some of them are, perhaps 20%.'

Other questions that had been posed within this section were about the use of theory to guide practice, Table 6.12(1); research findings, Table 6.12(2); occupational therapy activities, Table 6.12(5) and problem solving skills, Table 6.12(7). All elicited rather a wide spread of responses. A need to have had 'life experience' was rated highly by users, Table 6.12(9). One question within this section related to a knowledge of physical illnesses, Table 6.12(3), an issue that had arisen on a number of occasions during the Focus Group discussions. Comments from users suggested that the issue for them was to be taken seriously when they presented ailments of a possibly physical illness. Users were not concerned as such with mental health nurses not having a specific knowledge of physical illnesses but felt that they should at least take their complaints seriously and refer them on accordingly. As one user commented, 'when I first went into hospital I complained about tonsillitis, no one looked at my throat for two weeks and I ended up with a chest infection'. The student responses showed that they did not rate highly the importance of a knowledge base of physical illnesses, Table 6.13(3); although some did comment that 'you have got to know something about physical illnesses to do your job properly'.

The 'any other comments' question elicited very general comments that fitted into the following themes:

- Relevant and practical after care that is available at weekends.
- Empathy. The following verbatim quotes may make clear this issue, the first quote is from a user and the second from a nursing student. 'It is important to try and understand what it feels like to have a mental illness, then they may begin to treat you better.' 'Nurses should respect, empathise and value patients as individuals who have an illness or mental health problems. They should be perceived as unique individuals who need help and the nurse's role should be first and foremost to give that help and meet the needs of the patient.' These sentiments appear to be at the heart of the concerns of many users. Often it had been stated that it was an individual nurse who had acted as a friend and not the services per se that had been of greatest benefit to them.
- Promote independence. Some users had experienced the contradiction of being on a so-called rehabilitation ward only to find themselves locked out of their rooms, having to attend occupational therapy whether it was relevant or not and having to ask a member of staff if they could go into the kitchen that was usually locked.
- Manage the environment of care. As one user succinctly put it, 'I found smoking on the ward made the atmosphere stuffy and the tranquillisation by television a hindrance to social relations'.
- A need for a clearer role definition regarding therapeutic skills and practice as 'therapy is talked about enough but nurses need to be seen

doing therapeutic work. The nurse should not refer so much and take the therapeutic work on board in the ward, get involved more and don't let someone else do it. Whatever the psychiatric nurse does they need to be seen doing it'.

- Permanent staff. Less use of agency nurses and of the promoting of bank nursing: 'The lack of permanent staff on wards makes jobs for nurses difficult as regularly changing agency nurses often means that the burden falls on the permanent staff who are then overstretched and stressed and they do not have time to spend with patients. The patients lose out on proper care and attention. Short-term contract staff cannot feel involved and are more concerned about themselves and about their own jobs and futures'.

In summary, the biographical data does suggest that there are some notable differences between users and students. In relation to what a nurse should do, be and know, there is considerable convergence between the user and the student nurses' responses but there are also indecisive responses. The convergent and the divergent issues will be discussed in greater detail in the next chapter.

References

Department of Health 1989 Caring for people: community care into the next decade and beyond. Department of Health, London

Department of Health 1991 The health of the nation. The Stationary Office, London

Department of Health 1994a Working in partnership - report of the Mental Health Nursing Review Team. HMSO, London

McIver S 1991 An introduction to obtaining the views of users of health services. Kings Fund, London

Raphael W 1977 Osychiatric hospitals viewed by their patients. Kings Fund, London

Burnard P 1994 Keep it simple. Nursing Standard 8(34):41

Horwitz A 1983 The social construct of mental illness. Academy, New York

Strauss A, Corbin J 1988 Shaping a health care system. Jossey Bass, San Francisco

Handyside E, Heyman B 1994 Mental illness in the community: the role of voluntary and state agencies. In: Heyman B (ed) Researching user perspectives on community health care. Chapman and Hall, London

Pilgrim D, Rogers A 1993 Sociology of mental health and illness. OUP, Buckingham

National Statistic Office 2003 Census 2001. Online. Available: http://www.statistics.gov.uk/cci/nugget.asp?id=350 15

Department of Health 1994b The Allitt inquiry. HMSO, London

Editorial 1997 Nursing Standard 11(38):6

Chapter 7

Differing perspectives – divergence and convergence

INTRODUCTION

This chapter is an integration and analysis of the data obtained from the research. It identifies the different perspectives from a user and nursing position and considers how meaningful partnerships can be developed. Two distinct options are presented as a way forward and recommendations made in the context of government initiatives and proposed changes within mental health services. They are synthesised and discussed in the context of the research questions.

WHAT ARE THE VIEWS AND PERCEIVED NEEDS OF USERS OF MENTAL HEALTH SERVICES IN THE CONTEXT OF THE ROLE THAT USERS SEE MENTAL HEALTH NURSES FULFILLING?

A précis of the issues identified within the user literature indicates that the key concerns relate to individuality, choice, information, quality of care and the social and economic circumstances of their lives. There is no doubt that users are greatly concerned with issues of information provision within mental health services and the need for fully informed choice and negotiated health care. Users are not requesting expensive or unreasonable therapies or interventions, but are asking for rudimentary support that is provided in a compassionate manner when they are distressed and that they are treated as individuals and not reduced to mere illness entities. The social and economic context of their lives, the degree to which social conditions can contribute to, or exacerbate, mental health problems and how, as users, they can be realistically reintegrated into society are prominent issues of concern. The key findings from this research concur with the above. The Rank Order Exercise identified the following as the most important factors in terms of what nurses should 'do':

- Listen to users as individuals
- Show respect
- Boost confidence and independence
- Spend more time with users
- Manage aggression and show understanding.

In terms of what nurses should 'be' the following were the five top ranked issues:

- Friendly and human
- Sensitive and approachable
- Self aware and mature
- Non threatening
- Available/interested in nursing as a career.

The five top ranked issues as to what a nurse should 'know' were:
1) More about medical and physical problems
2) Medication and its effects
3) Experiences of life
4) Communication skills
5) Talking therapies/problem solving approaches.

The data from Stage 2 confirms these issues from a user perspective and primarily indicates that there is a gap between how users have defined their needs and what they actually experience in practice.

Information provision and choice

The research identifies the importance for users of receiving information if they are to engage in a truly collaborative approach to care, and nurses are perceived as being in an ideal position to be proactive information givers. However, from the views expressed by users and the ratings given in the questionnaires about how helpful nurses are in providing information, there is little evidence to support that this happens regularly or consistently in practice. Hogg (1994) suggests that information can help people to use services better, improve their health by following suggestions or advice, manage their situation and make choices and decisions, thus enabling people to move from a dependency or passive mode of functioning to a more active one that is more consistent with working in partnership. This can be a process of empowerment that some professionals may find very threatening since they may have to let go of their positions of power and work closer *with* service users rather then *for* them from the position of professionals who often think that they know best. The user participants saw themselves as clients with legitimate expectations and rights. They expressed their need for help at a vulnerable time. Their vulnerability may impose limitations to the way they live their lives but does not mean that they forfeit, more generally, their rights and responsibilities as adults. To be given information is an important part of boosting one's confidence, of maintaining control of one's own life and of being respected by others as well as being placed in a position to contribute in an informed manner to the decision making process. One cannot begin to enter into partnership relationships without having access to relevant information. It is clear that users see nurses as having a central role to play in the provision of information, since they are the ones with whom users have the most contact, but in practice users felt that nurses were not providing the information required. Studies by Hall and Dornan (1988) and Lovell (1995) have consistently found that, when specific questions are asked, users express dissatisfaction with the information that they receive about their illness diagnosis and treatment. Users identified repeatedly that they want improved information about treatment options, services that are available and facts concerning drugs used within psychiatry. A recurring theme was that users felt that there was not enough detail given on the side effects of medication. As a result they did not know whether some of the symptoms that they experienced were side effects or not, which added to their feelings of anxiety and distress. One of the five top ranked issues in Stage 1 of this research in relation to what a nurse should 'know' was about medication and its effects. This was also reflected in comments expressed on the questionnaires in Stage 2.

Campbell (1996) suggests that 'for many service users information giving and caring have taken on an equal importance'. He further reports that over the last decade there certainly has been an increase in the amount of information that is available and for nurses he suggests that

> '... they must face up to the challenge of themselves knowing enough about treatments to give information on demand. They should become proactive in disseminating information to those in their care. It is no longer acceptable for questions about treatments to be side-stepped or for mental health workers to refer people to the local reference library for more details and to pretend they are providing a good service'.

To enable users to maintain control over their own lives it is important that they be given proper information about the practices and expectations, their rights and complaint procedures within mental health services. It is clear that users feel that nurses have a central role in this when engaging with them and that nurses should be willing to act as a supporter, putting the interests of users first. Providing information can also be part of a process of cementing relationships that can help to dispel feelings of 'us and them', thus enhancing co-operation and leading to more effective partnership working.

The Code of Practice on Openness in the NHS (National Health Service Executive 1995 p2) stated almost ten years ago that, 'because the NHS is a public service, it should be open about its activities and plans,' and furthermore it identified four core aims as to ensure that people:

1. Have access to available information about the services provided by the NHS, the cost of these services, quality standards and performance

against targets;

2. Are provided with explanations about proposed service changes and have an opportunity to influence decisions;

3. Are aware of the reasons for decisions and actions affecting their own treatment;

4. Know what information is available, where and how they can get it.

But other than publishing the name of an individual who has the responsibility for the Code, the role of the nurse with regard to information giving was not mentioned. Users' experiences indicate that a structured system whereby the nurse on the ward is given responsibility and accountability for the provision of information is not generally being seen to operate. Some users expressed cynicism about information that they were provided with. This reflected concern that information can be limited in its reliability, by how it originates and the agenda it is aspiring to address. Many users still feel that they are expected to take on the sick role, defer to professionals and take the prescribed medication. Thus, it is important to consider the context and the perspective in which the provision of information takes place. Users stated that they and their families need reliable information to help them to understand their illness and difficulties and they require clarification of what type of treatment and help is available. For nurses to have a proper role in the provision of information to service users, it must be within a professional structure and they must be accountable for the information they give. It must be within a framework of openness and impartiality with no hidden agendas. Users see information in the context of the quality of the care provided. The provision of information should be based on real alternatives and choice and be an expression of a real commitment to collaboration and partnership in care.

Quality of care and therapeutic interventions

The therapeutic interventions that users see as being of greatest benefit in satisfying their needs are social skills training and interventions that help them with everyday difficulties such as housing issues and being occupied in a useful and worthwhile manner that has relevance to their life in society. Interventions that involve nurses spending time with users, listening and problem solving, are of high priority. Therapy such as counselling is appreciated by users who see it as a way nurses could spend planned, purposeful and structured time with them. A study by McGonagle and Gentle (1996) suggests that there exists a lack of partnership on choice of therapy, particularly given the emphasis on group work, which 86% found unhelpful. They report that users felt uncomfortable, fearful and unable to cope in group assessment situations; in addition users stated that the activities and subject matter of group work were at times totally inappropriate. Inappropriate use of groups can heighten users' feelings that they are not in control, as groups can strip people's individuality, create a forum where there is pressure to conform and enhance the power of the leader. This research also found that users' experiences of groups were that they were not always appropriate in addressing their needs and were merely ways of attempting to keep people occupied. The issues discussed were often perceived as trivial and mundane, not of any real concern to users, and the facilitation was often lacking any structure. Properly run, groups might have been beneficial for exploring and working through their real problems but that was not their experience. The answers on the questionnaire relating to nurses having the ability to run groups effectively were unsupported but some positive comments did relate to groups which had addressed day-to-day problems and social skills training.

It is important to reflect on the negative feedback from users about groups in terms of wider issues. It indicates the danger of superimposing therapeutic interventions onto a service that, in so many ways, is still embedded in institutional culture. Both the need for the therapy and the outcomes may be distorted by the culture within which it operates. Nurses must have appropriate skills and feel competent in their own abilities if they are to be able to assess individuals' needs proficiently and to facilitate those needs within a therapeutic setting if such therapy is to prove useful to users. The required skills and how they are assessed will be determined by what outcomes the service is trying to achieve, how clearly those outcomes are defined and communicated and what changes are made in practice to achieve these outcomes. However, a medical model of psychiatry is still the dominant culture. The emphasis is upon chemical changes in the brain, the identification of signs and symptoms, diagnosis that is a medical definition of the problem and an over-dependence upon medication. As a result of that dominant culture, change is not only slow but also in some areas reactionary. Reflecting back, the 1968 review of mental health nursing alluded to the need for nursing to become more therapeutic in its vocation, to engage in research and to distinguish good practices. The review saw the role of the nurse as 'diverse' but the emphasis was on keeping the users occupied and to that extent one might conclude that group work does achieve the determined outcome.

Users placed much emphasis on the need for higher quality care than that which they were receiving and it is in this context that the effectiveness or not of therapeutic interventions, which users had experienced in practice, were judged. The quality of care was seen to depend to a great extent upon the personality and ability of the individual nurse to deliver, and the effectiveness of their skills were seen to be dependent upon their commitment to their work. Wright (1989) describes a hapless situation whereby health professionals are expected to take on the facilitation of therapies of many sorts without any substantive training whatsoever. More often than not these people are young and enthusiastic nurses, but unfortunately they are lacking in experience, knowledge, confidence and sadly as a result are practically set up to fail. Therapeutic intervention should be considered as an essential part of mental health service provision and it is the responsibility of service providers to ensure that such services are set up first and foremost to be therapeutic. However, users do not always experience the outcomes as therapeutically effective. If the task of running therapeutic groups is delegated to the least qualified and experienced, it is not surprising that users are indicating its failure. What we may have in the service is the construction of a therapeutic façade perpetuated by either the service not giving a clear direction on desired outcomes or ignorance on behalf of the more senior staff, with a lack of will or interest to see such schemes succeed.

Users were more positive specifically about counselling. They appreciated the opportunity for one-to-one contact but again indicated that for it to be most effective nurses should be educated and trained in counselling theory and skills. Counselling offers nursing a more structured and disciplined way in which to spend time with users and encourages a move away from the notion that still appears to be prevalent in nursing, that time spent talking is not the best use of time, especially with those diagnosed with a psychotic illness. For users, quality of care was synonymous with interpersonal relationships and the effectiveness of care would be determined by the interpersonal skills of the nurse. Users saw counselling as a way for nurses to operate effective interpersonal skills in a structured framework. However, users also indicated that the theory and practice of counselling was not the only measure of what would make counselling useful for them. They also felt that nurses should have an appropriate empathetic attitude, which is a more intangible characteristic but nonetheless fundamental to nurses treating those in their care with dignity and compassion. Both the 1968 and the 1994 reviews of mental health nursing recognised the need for effective interpersonal skills and appropriate attitudes and most nursing courses now place interpersonal skills as a vital part of nursing. Yet this research shows that users felt that nurses were not adopting the appropriate empathetic attitudes or using effective interpersonal skills consistently in practice.

Users also emphasised that an important indicator of the quality of their care, their interpersonal relationships with nurses and the effectiveness of any specific therapeutic intervention, is whether they are listened to. Listening skills were rated highly by users in Stage 1 and commented upon on a number of occasions throughout the study. The findings in Stage 2 show that the students highly rated the need to listen to users, but the users' views suggest that nurses are not always prepared to listen to them. Listening to users and hearing what they have to say with an open and honest attitude is seen as an essential aspect of the nurse's role, again probably an obvious role expectation but one not always experienced in practice. Many users felt that not being listened to reflected the negative and stereotyped view of the mentally ill, particularly those that have been diagnosed with a psychotic illness. This view holds that the mentally ill cannot be expected to show any real insight about what is best for them and therefore their opinions and ideas are not really listened to and are regularly disparaged. Sheldon (1997) concerning seven admissions that she had experienced states that, 'The reason I took so long to sort it all out, why I had so many readmissions and why I suffered so much was because no one really talked to me. They did things for me and to me but not with me'. She also describes her experience as a service user relating to an incident involving sanitary towels in a plastic bag that were forcibly confiscated by a nurse. Her attempt to resist their confiscation resulted in five nurses descending and manhandling her into a side-room, injecting her with medication and then leaving her in a state of confusion. The plastic bag had been the focus of concern as a potential suicide risk, yet no one chose to simply ask her for the bag.

The Mental Health Foundation (1997) in its report found that users were very positive about talking treatments. The reasons given for this were that users felt that they were being given the opportunity to be listened to and understood; they were treated as a whole person; they were able to express their feelings and gain understanding of their problems and hence feel more in control of their lives. However, despite this evidence there are detractors of talking treatments (Masson 1988, Weldon 1997) who not only question their effectiveness but also suggest that they can be oppressive and manipulative. Perhaps more research is needed in this area but such 'black and white' positions do not further an understanding of those interventions nor take users' views into consideration. Again, the effectiveness of therapies must be considered within the context in which they are being practised. There is always the potential for therapies to be used to manipulate and control the vulnerable. Effective outcomes depend on the skill of those practising the therapy, whether or not they receive clinical supervision, whether they are able to conduct an accurate assessment of the individual's needs and offer proper choice and whether they achieve willing collaboration and participation. Users in this research expressed the need for more talking therapeutic interventions and for time to be allocated for that to actually happen. Their responses reflect the consistent emphasis that users placed on structured therapies that involved one-to-one contact with nurses. These findings match some of the findings of Jackson and Stevenson (1998) who also found that what users wanted from mental health nurses was time, emotional commitment and knowledge to help them explore and understand their distress and subsequent difficulties.

The idea of having an identified named nurse to turn to was regarded as desirable and identified as beneficial by users. However, concerns were expressed about the named person actually being available or contactable when needed, which indicates that it is questionable whether or not the concept is really understood by nurses in terms of the full responsibility of the role. Although there is support for named nursing in theory, with the idea of the named nurse being embedded in the many policy guidelines, it does not appear to be transferred regularly into practice. Staff shortages may be one variable that has to be considered. According to Dooley (1999) continuity of care is a key issue in named nursing but a shortage of staff is the major detriment to maintaining the named nurse. Furthermore, Dooley suggests that the management of care on the wards is ambiguous, the duty rotas are not very effective and the potential of the night staff is unrealised. The 1968 review of mental health nursing focused on staffing levels as a necessary factor in achieving outcomes. The need had been identified for more support staff to relieve nurses of non-nursing duties and for an increase in staffing levels to enable nurses to spend more time with users in order to develop genuine therapeutic relationships. The 1994 mental health nursing review gave greater emphasis to the issues identified in the 1968 review, but also stressed the need for the development of the role of nurses as key workers/care coordinators within the Care Programme Approach, supervised discharge and the provision of information to service users. In this research, users acknowledged that the named nurse and the care coordinator system are positive developments in terms of having an identified person to turn to who monitors and coordinates their care, but they suggested that in the majority of cases it is not happening in practice. If it is to be of any real value to service users then certain changes must take place to enable the strategy to happen. Again the focus must be on meeting the needs of users. Campbell (1996 p12) has expressed concern that there may be a danger of moving towards a culture of 'nursing by appointment only' and hence there is a need to be aware of that possible scenario.

The findings from the second stage did not indicate that users were greatly dissatisfied with the staffing levels experienced. Again, the emphasis was on the quality of interaction when staff were available and the priority that should be given to this. Unfortunately, users see the role of the nurse as, fundamentally, one that is predominately concerned with administration, the giving out of medicine, custodial and only therapeutic when time permits and not when the need arises or as a high priority. Nurses were also seen as disempowered to the extent that they are controlled by the decisions of psychiatrists. The report produced by The Mental Health Act Commission and The Sainsbury Centre for Mental Health (MHAC/SCMH) (1997 p1) states in the summary of their key findings from a one-day visit to 309 acute psychiatric wards in 1997 that the wards were generally found to be adequately staffed by nurses who regularly worked on the wards and were familiar with them; there was also a reasonable proportion of qualified staff. Thus in a situation where staff shortages have not been identified the question is, how do nurses actually spend their time? The MHAC/SCMH concluded that many of the difficulties observed on their visits related to proper procedures and the lack of time spent by nursing staff with service users and that the situation could be improved with management attention. They recommended that there was a need for clear operational policies, effective leadership and support to help nurses to maintain their motivation and commitment to their work. Alden's (1978) research into treatment environments and user improvement concluded that the clinical areas that have greater user–staff interaction displayed more user improvement. Users are still saying that this is what they want but their experience of mental health services is that user–nurse interaction is not a priority on wards and users feel nurses are often unapproachable, while nurses profess that they do not have sufficient time to spend with users. The responses within the questionnaires in this research revealed that being approachable was also rated highly in terms of what nurses should 'be'. Users' comments made clear that, based on their experiences of personal responses from individual nurses, approachability was determined by certain personal characteristics and attitudes. However, users also clearly felt that the system did not prioritise their real needs and was organised in such a way to make it easy for nurses not to be approachable; nor did the system appear to value, nurture and reward the attitudes that users felt were important. Outcomes must be determined by proper research of what works for users and the priorities for nursing practice must be established to achieve those outcomes. The task for managers and nurses is to maintain their focus on and motivation around those outcomes in their day-to-day work and not to be driven by other agendas.

It is in relation to their views of appropriate attitudes that users judge the quality and effectiveness of any intervention. For example, physical restraint was seen by users as being potentially an intervention that could be reassuring and protective but often experienced negatively as being an uncaring and an overpowering ordeal. Users saw managing aggression as part of the role of the nurse and expressed views that it needs to be done much more tactfully and sensitively. The findings from the literature reviewed suggest a need for a change to more positive attitudes towards users. In both stages of the research, users identified issues relating to the need for nurses to be much more effective in their interpersonal skills. Views were expressed that nurses should be sensitive, compassionate and approachable and be good listeners, to hear what users are saying and not to dismiss their views as inconsequential. Users wanted nurses to be friendly, humane and kind but not patronising, this was expressed in the context of users feeling that they were not being responded to with equality as human beings, an issue that constantly arose. They did not want to be differentiated into 'another' category that merely takes account of their illness. Empathy was another intangible quality that users felt nurses should exhibit, a word that is used frequently by nurses, but its meaning was often lost. Users felt that age and life experiences, including being mental health service users, were factors which might positively affect a nurse's ability to empathise and that these issues should be incorporated into recruitment policy. Another attribute that users felt nurses should have was to be genuinely interested in nursing as a career, which would be likely to underpin positive motivation and thus determine attitudes.

Concerns about nurses' knowledge

The data from the questionnaire does not put a specific nursing knowledge base high on the agenda and there was some cynicism expressed about the benefits of education for improving the nurse–user relationship, in terms of the extent to which education is able to impart qualities of 'personality'. As one user commented:

> 'Nurses are very important, I grant you in our well being. Even so, I have to be convinced that any more education is likely to succeed. The care, patience and understanding that they should have taken in with their mother's milk have often gone by the wayside. Why bother pouring in more education until nursing gets some of those qualities back? What would it be founded on?'

However, users do identify the need for nurses to have a working knowledge relating to interpersonal and social needs and about medication. To recap on the knowledge base of nursing that was perceived as important by users in the Rank Order exercise:

- More about medical and physical problems
- Medication and its effects
- Life experience
- Communication skills
- Talking therapies/problem solving approaches.

During the Focus Group discussions users clearly identified the need for mental health nurses to have a solid working knowledge of medicines and physical ailments. The issue of physical ailments was identified as being an issue of concern and spoken about a great deal in the group discussions. Users expressed concern that their reporting of physical complaints was not taken seriously and often dismissed or reinterpreted as symptom of their mental illness. Some of the students recognised and agreed with this belief: 'Some idea of physical illnesses is important so that patients do not have to go to general wards for simple things, one needs to know that a person is unwell as they are often accused of putting it on'. Another student commented that 'Due to the training, knowledge of physical illness within mental health nursing is very limited, this could constitute a danger to the client at times especially when basic biological and physiological knowledge is not held by the nurse'. Some users reported the difficulty of obtaining an aspirin for a simple headache as being a major hurdle in itself and it was usually easier to go to the nearest shop, but this depended on if they were open and on the time of day.

The responses to the questionnaire also indicated that users felt nurses needed to know more about medical and physical problems, and again, some of the comments suggested that what users meant by that response was that they felt that they were not being taken seriously when they raised their medical problems with nurses. The fact that users could not get their needs met in respect of physical ailments was a useful tangible example on which they could focus, which was really a reflection of the problems of poor interpersonal relationships, communication and not being respected as an individual, rather than solely about nurses not having sufficient knowledge. Nurses' knowledge of the medication used for treating 'mental illnesses' was raised primarily within the context of users being given information.

In the context of nurses having a knowledge base for the purpose of functioning as 'autonomous practitioners and professionals', these concepts were not the focus of users' concerns. However, it was indicated that nurses should not adopt an *ad hoc* approach to their work, which should be underpinned by research, and nurses should be prepared to accept responsibility and function proactively. Users attached much importance to nurses being knowledgeable in relation to interpersonal skills and communication skills. It is unambiguous that users placed tangible skills on a bedrock of nurses having appropriate attitudes.

Social and economic support

Many of the complaints expressed by users about their treatment on wards and within the community centred on the negative stereotype image of mentally ill people. Their diagnosis became a problem in itself, with the negative image reflected back on to them through their treatment by others and by institutions. Being defined in terms of a negative stereotype had practical consequences on their lives in relation to their social and economic existence. Users wanted nurses to disregard stereotypes and prejudice, to get to know them as individuals and to see them as people not cases. Furthermore, they wanted meaningful help to deal with those problems and felt that nurses had a role in helping to dispel a negative image of mental illness. However, users expressed concern that their actual experience of conduct within mental health services involved a perpetuation of the stereotype, both in terms of their one-to-one contact and the priorities of mental health services and how the services were organised. Thus users were asking not to be embedded into a medical model of psychiatry or to be treated as stereotypes by nurses and other health care professionals. They wanted nurses to provide practical help to overcome the problems in the wider community that they were experiencing as a result of their mental illness diagnosis and which could be as concerning as the effects of their suffering itself. Users wanted nurses to help maintain their contact with the wider community in a practical way by helping them to obtain meaningful skills and to be able to operate effectively at a social and economic level in the community.

Users expressed that often the help that they were given through occupational therapy was meaningless and unhelpful for the reality of the world with which they have to cope. It did not help them get a job or build and maintain social relationships. Users did not want nurses to ignore this issue but to help them deal with it, which is a very important factor in boosting confidence and independence. These findings indicate that social integration and unemployment are major difficulties for users. A report by Meltzer et al (1995 p139) focused upon economic activity and social functioning of adults with a diagnosed psychiatric disorder. It indicated that 'only 4 in 10 adults with a psychotic disorder were working compared with 6 in 10 of those with a neurotic disorder and 7 in 10 unaffected by a mental disorder'. Financially, they also appeared to be at a disadvantage since the 'median weekly, gross, individual income was more than a third less than those without a psychiatric disorder'. There are great difficulties for users in becoming fully integrated into society since with a reduced income and meagre job prospects it is easy to see why those with a history of 'mental illness' might remain on the margins of society. This highlights the actual task of rehabilitation with the aim to return people to the labour market. It is likely that employer attitudes will be informed and influenced by the negative stereotypes of the mentally ill that generally prevail in society and which are perpetuated by the media. This would have the effect of discouraging any potential employer taking what they perceive to be a risk in employing someone with a history of mental health problems.

There was some conflicting evidence from the different stages of this research regarding the involvement of family and significant others in treatment and care. This may be due to the fact that the research indicated that frequently users did not have a close-knit circle of family and friends. However, Rose (1996 p18) reports from her research that 'it is clear that people with mental health problems want more contact with family, friends and community organisations'. From the evidence of her findings she drew up a league table of the interviewees' preferences for the involvement of different groups. This also gives an indication of the extent of negative interaction faced by users in the wider community:

1. Friends – the most valued group with which users felt they could share their experiences and receive understanding.
2. Church – the personal and social side of this experience as well as the religious one.
3. Family – both positive and negative feelings were expressed.
4. Community organisations (e.g. Citizens Advice Bureau, law centres, adult education) – the social side of the interaction was important as well as the practical help and on 'the whole they felt they were being treated with respect and dignity'.
5. Local community (people in pubs, clubs and shops) – the commonest feelings about the local community were a mixture of good and bad experiences.
6. Work colleagues – not many worked but those who did had mixed feelings as to how they were received.
7. Neighbours – the predominant experience was negative.
8. Housing agencies – perceived as offhand, disrespectful and unhelpful.
9. Department of Social Security – 'they treat you as a mental case'.
10. Work supervisors – those who had them found them difficult.
11. The police – interviewees felt the police to be particularly prejudiced and contact especially negative.

It might be helpful if the stereotype of being 'mentally ill' is challenged directly. Nurses and other health care professionals need to take on the issue, discuss it with users and work through it together as a problem that they will have to face within the community. Users need help to achieve skills to deal with the negative situations that arise, turn them to their best advantage and achieve more positive outcomes in terms of their life generally. For nurses to take this forward they must be aware of their own prejudices and perspectives and how these can play a part in their dealings with those that use mental health services. To fulfil this role effectively nurses need both the skills to communicate and facilitate but also the appropriate attitude and to have a developed level of self-awareness. It is quite clear that users do want nurses to help them to address the significant issues that they have to deal with in their everyday lives.

HOW DO STUDENT NURSES PERCEIVE THEIR FUTURE ROLE GIVEN THE CHANGES IN NURSE PREPARATION?

It has been suggested by Jackson and Stevenson (1998 p31) 'that there are many conflicting ideas about what mental health nurses actually do and what they ought to do'. Reflecting upon the literature, the 1968 review of mental health nursing expressed concern that nursing should become much more therapeutic. In 1982 a new syllabus of training was introduced with nurses being expected to be aware of a wide range of social and psychological issues in the causation and treatment of mental distress. The 1994 review equally stressed the notion of therapeutic relationships and the need for nursing to be more accountable for its actions. The 1990s were very much influenced by the raising of the baseline pre-registration qualification from certificate level to diploma and degree level. This has been done in an attempt to enhance the professional standing of nursing and to generate research that could enhance the quality of care within the context of evidence-based practice. Discussion continues to take place regarding the aspiration to an all-graduate profession that is sufficiently rewarding and explicit in a clinical career, but England lags behind the rest of the UK, mainly due to the difficulties in recruiting sufficient numbers who would meet the entrance criteria for degree level preparation.

The data from the students verifies that they placed a high value on education and research. They perceived themselves as being different from their predecessors because of being exposed to a higher education and as more reflective and critical of their clinical experience and the quality of care that they had observed. They provided many written comments regarding the importance of knowledge, the need for research to inform practice and for nurses to take on more responsibility, to be more accountable and to develop in a true professional manner.

The issues that the students identified relating to their future role can quite clearly be synthesised into the concept of a 'therapeutic agent' with the service user at the centre of their work. In peripheral discussions there was consistency in recognising the need to engage with users in a structured way in endeavouring to identify priorities and facilitate problem solving. The students had identified the following during the Rank Order Exercise regarding what a nurse should 'do':

- Listen to users as individuals
- Boost confidence and independence
- Spend more time with users
- Show respect
- Develop support networks.

Regarding what a nurse should 'be':

- Self aware and mature/sensitive and approachable
- Advocate and agent of change
- Competent independent practitioner
- Empathic person first then a nurse
- Available.

The data from the questionnaires indicated that nurses recognised and perceived their role as important in improving communication with users, providing relevant information, treating users more as individuals with individual needs and abilities and engaging with them in meaningful activities that have a bearing on their everyday needs and lifestyles. In Stage 2, 88% (n=176) of students selected 'being approachable', as the most important in terms of what a nurse should 'be'. The everyday needs of users tended to come to the fore, with the students acknowledging the need to engage in confidence building, promotion of independence and social skill training. However, concern was expressed that they did not get any effective training in relation to this latter point. The need to address issues regarding housing, retraining and realistic employment options was seen as part of the role of the nurse within the context of rehabilitation.

Support and supervision

An issue that was highlighted in relation to how students saw their future role was whether or not they would be able to maintain their integrity once they were qualified and became part of a team with established values, norms and a culture of its own. In this context, some appreciated the need for continued support and supervision as a way of reviewing clinical work and their own personal development. Martin (1984) commenting on nursing during the 1960s and 1970s posed the question: 'How is it that institutions established to care for those in need could have allowed them to be neglected, treated with callousness and even deliberate cruelty?' Part of his answer to that question was that nurses who felt under-valued and unsupported themselves vented their frustrations on patients. Similarly, findings from this research found that there was much concern on the part of the student nurses about how they would maintain their integrity to deliver user-centred quality care and continue to put theory into practice as newly qualified nurses. During the Focus Group discussions and from comments within the questionnaires, students on the basis of their experience of clinical practice expressed the difficulty of change. They voiced doubts about their ability to act as 'agents of change' in the face of the status quo. Many students recognised the need for research to guide their practice and saw it as a way of influencing and changing practice. However, some students had met with disparaging and cynical attitudes, rather than support, towards research whilst on their placements when they were informed that they would soon learn the reality of their role by experience. Student discussion groups were seen as very supportive in the face of these attitudes and students felt that continuing support is vital when they qualify.

The students saw supervision as a way of supporting nurses to fulfil their role, to develop and challenge the traditional theories and explanations of psychiatry, culture and science. Supervision was regarded as a key to successful change and in promoting effective clinical practice. However, clinical supervision is an issue that has been on the nursing agenda for some time (Butterworth & Faugier 1992, Department of Health 1994), and has been very slow to become established in a meaningful way. Supervision is a reflective process that aims to promote self-examination, evaluation and review and has the potential to enhance practice and sustain staff morale. Van Ooijen (1994) acknowledges that it may have the potential for the development of nursing but warns of the dangers, given the traditional culture of nursing, and contends that it could be used in a punitive way as a control mechanism. He suggests that 'admitting to mistakes or errors of judgement has not been the culture of nursing. Rather than help people to reflect and learn from their experiences nursing has tended to punish those who make errors by disciplining them'. Supervision should enable the practitioner to discuss what has been done, what they felt worked or did not work, to explore obstructions and options and also to give the nurse the opportunity to off-load some of their emotional baggage. Nevertheless, the question, 'Is the cultural climate of nursing truly ready to take on board such openness and honesty?' needs to be answered, not only by words but also by actions. The Mental Health Nursing Review team reported in 1994 that 'if mental health nurses are to meet the challenges of the future, they should have access to skilled clinical supervision ... and managers may well need to restructure services to make it a reality'. One cannot expect to find a panacea within the notion of supervision and it needs to be evaluated in terms of its effectiveness. In an attempt to address that issue, a clinical supervision evaluation project funded by the Department of Health and the Scottish Home and Health Department, in conjunction with the University of Manchester (1996), made the following recommendations:

1. Progress already made in providing clinical supervision be maintained and taken further given the support reported by participants in this study.
2. Trusts provide sufficient initial training and continued support for supervisors.
3. Employers examine further the evidence associated between personal perceptions of physical fitness, burnout and psychological well being.
4. Research is continued to assess longer-term impact of clinical supervision on the workforce through second generation studies.
5. The focused nature of clinical supervision and its emphasis on good practice and the well being of the workforce should be recognised by purchasers and providers: seen as 'good practice' by both and written into contract specifications.

Sadly, this simply has not happened.

Therapeutic interventions

The importance of communication skills has been recognised, and counselling specifically was identified as a way of offering a structured approach to engage with users. Communication skills and counselling were seen as core skills and both rated very highly by the students. Counselling was seen as a means by which planned time could be allocated with the opportunity for problem solving in a structured manner and the establishment of a meaningful therapeutic relationship. It appears that counselling is on the syllabus of training and education of nurses and is being promoted and grasped as a useful therapeutic means of intervention. The need to involve family members in the care process was identified, rated highly and seen as a role for nurses, but not elaborated upon within a context of a theoretical framework, for example family therapy or working in partnership. Despite the need being acknowledged to involve family members, the exact manner or purpose remains rather elusive other than by providing support to the user when they are discharged.

There was very little mention of any other interventions other than having responsibility for administering medication. Social skills training is seen as relevant, but the students did not experience such programmes in practice or as part of their own preparation for practice. Cognitive behavioural programmes or the use of electroconvulsive therapy (ECT) were seldom mentioned.

Nurses' role in the social and economic integration of users

Care and support programmes that involve helping people to manage their lives more effectively, for example social skills, job opportunities and housing, are clearly to the fore in terms of how the role of nursing was perceived by the student nurses. They did not rate very highly the effectiveness of nurses in dispelling a negative image of mental illness and, from some of the comments that were made, it does not appear to be clear how exactly this role could be achieved. It was understood by the student nurses that the stigma that is attached to people with a diagnosis of a 'mental illness' can make things worse by creating a barrier to employment and integration into economic and social activities that in turn can lead to isolation and a downward spiral of lack of confidence and low self esteem. It was acknowledged that this could influence how others relate to users and adversely affect the overall quality of their lives. The student nurses raised as a key point the importance of not reducing users to a diagnostic label.

From the responses of the students, the training and education of nurses does not prepare them for taking on a role of helping users with their social and economic needs, which users had said were not met, although the students acknowledged that nurses were well placed to have such a role. Poverty and inadequate housing are particularly common amongst people with mental health problems. Even though those matters are high priorities for users, they are often overlooked by professionals, who focus mainly on treatment and therapy and tend to ignore users' social and economic needs. Practical social care and treatment is required to help users stay out of hospitals and help them to remain integrated into society, otherwise there is a danger of leaving people isolated, lonely and with no sense of purpose to their lives. Kammerling and O'Connor (1993) also inform us that 'the association between socio-economic status and admission to hospitals for mental illness has been recognised for more than fifty years'. They suggest that unemployment rates are a useful marker for socio-economic deprivation and this has profound resource implications for mental health service provisions in areas with high unemployment. If this is not taken into account then those with serious mental health problems will be further disadvantaged. Nolan and Clancy (1995) report that there is a wealth of literature relating to social functioning from a professional carers' perspective but very little from a user's position. In an attempt to address this situation they engaged in a study that involved thirty users to ascertain the nature and value of the social networks in which they were currently involved. They concluded that:

'Despite having participated in a variety of rehabilitation interventions, these clients remained insecure and lacking in confidence. They had few friends beyond members of their immediate family and were generally leading lonely, friendless existences without the capacity to establish new relationships. Mental health nurses may best meet their needs by helping to sustain existing relationships and using them at all levels of therapeutic intervention'.

Within this research the student nurses highly rated the importance of maintaining contact for users within the locality, and of involving and working with families and significant others. How this will translate into future practice remains to be seen since this is another issue that has been on the health care agenda for a long time and to which many reports and research findings have drawn specific attention (Blom-Cooper et al 1995, Rogers et al 1993).

Administrative duties and time spent with users

The student nurses acknowledged that the role of the nurse encompasses administrative duties but it was often expressed that there was too much paperwork. Their clinical experiences led them to believe that there is a danger of paper and administrative work taking priority over spending time with and listening to users. They recognised that this could lead to a failure in care. As one student commented:

'nurse–patient interaction is very important in understanding patients problems, but time is so limited due to the importance given to administrative work, it takes on a higher priority. I think that it is about covering your back'.

So although nurses consistently recognise that there is a need to spend quality time with users, many students found that their experiences on the wards showed them that this is often compromised in the need to meet administrative deadlines. Gijbels and Burnard (1995) found that senior clinical staff usually do much of the administrative work while it is left to the inexperienced, newly or untrained staff to develop therapeutic relationships. It is essential that the most clinically able and experienced nurses learn to delegate some administrative duties and/or, in reviewing skill mixes, employ more clerical workers if administrative duties are too great. Nurses are being educated and trained at immense cost to fulfil a different role, which is to build relationships with users and help to address their needs. This is regarded as a core function of mental health nursing and the system of care must be managed in a manner that allows this to actually happen.

Attitudes and values

Sundeen et al (1985) contend that nurses cannot begin to understand the private world of service users unless they understand their own private world; that is, their feelings, attitudes, beliefs and values. To enable nurses to fulfil their role it is recognised that self-awareness is an essential element to any therapeutic relationship. The importance of this is the ability for nurses to be able to empathise with those in their care. This was an issue that emerged on a number of occasions and the students gave it the top ranking in the Rank Order Exercise and also rated it highly in their response to the questionnaire with 72% (n=144) rating it as very important. Rolfe (1990), who investigated therapeutic attitudes in psychiatric settings, draws attention to 'attitudes' as educational outcomes, and asks: 'what is it that constitutes desirable attitudes in the nurse?' He concludes that, 'in part, this meant those attitudes which, when held by the nurse, were found to be therapeutic to the patient'. An extensive review of the literature, which he undertook, revealed three such attitudes to be empathy, genuineness and respect. Those concepts are not new and have been written about a great deal. They have been identified by Rogers (1951) and Egan (1998) and many others as essential to any therapeutic relationship. The students mentioned these concepts as essential to practice but also questioned their application in the provision of care. Whether it is possible to teach or train someone to acquire such qualities is questionable and perhaps much more emphasis should be placed on trying to identify such traits at selection interviews. Close monitoring of such variables throughout nursing courses, during clinical practice and at annual appraisals for qualified nurses could take place in an attempt to maintain and promote such values in enabling nurses to be true to their perceived role.

A concern of major importance to the student nurses was, what happens to nurses' values as they gain more experience and enter fully into nursing practice with bona fide intentions? That concern is supported by Bergin and Soloman (1994) and Carkhuff et al (1968) who found that, although on commencing training prospective care workers functioned at a higher level than the typical lay person, soon after the completion of their course that level had dropped considerably. Farley and Hendry (1992) also identified a process of virtual metamorphosis from the enthusiastic and challenging student to the conformist qualified member of a team. This is a process that is incremental in nature and eventually succeeds in transforming the student to comply with the rules and norms of the service. The danger in this is that the desire and pressure to become part of a culture that is not necessarily in the users' best interest will not only be perpetuated but can also serve as a brake on any innovative developments and practice that should be at the heart of professional nursing. Martin (1984) reminds us that 'one must not forget that for creativity to be effective it has to gain a secure base in the actual working group and the bedrock on which the quality of care depends consists of staff and the ethics which motivate and guide them'. The following quote by a student nurse encapsulates the above issues:

'There is a wide gulf between what we are taught at college and real life on the ward. It would be very easy to fall into the smoking and reading magazines type shift work, which is perpetuated by some staff. Students have a hard time reconciling theory with being accepted by the ward staff, that is, not rocking the boat or being too enthusiastic and pushy on behalf of patients. It is hard to rise above the constant sea of cynicism that trained staff are drowning in'.

The students implied that contentment with a medical model of psychiatry appears to prevail as a dominant characteristic of the majority of nurses that they had worked with.

Compassion and kindness were words that had generated a lot of discussion by the student nurses. They recognised these concepts as important but they were not rated as highly as might have been expected, although, as mentioned previously, that may have been due to the problems in operationalising the words, which many of the written comments suggested. There was some concern that kindness could take on a patronising form. Nolan (1990) interestingly cites Edward Jorden (1569–1632) a physician who wrote about hysteria and suggested that, 'medicine had nothing to offer the sufferer, but that hysteria could be relieved by the ministration of a kind person'. Edward Jorden also established the criteria that attached to successful care. Those were the intangible qualities of sympathy, understanding, to be part of a welcoming community and that the person's understanding and consent to any intervention should be sought prior to treatment. The findings from this research show that those issues are of major significance to users and, even though they are on the mental health agenda, are yet so slow to be grasped and acted upon. How can we learn from failures of care? A 'bad apple' explanation is too simplistic and as Martin (1984 p242) had suggested 'in a hospital ward it is virtually impossible for one person to behave unprofessionally on more than one or two occasions without other staff and patients getting to know'. He further comments upon the power of the working group and its ability to influence the standard of care that is provided.

The concept of 'hero innovators' who could singlehandedly change the system has long been exposed as a myth (Georgiades & Phillimore 1975, Prail & Baldwin 1988) yet such eagerness for change continues to be expressed by newcomers to nursing, as these findings show. Perhaps the current reorganisation in the education of nurses and the health service generally may bring with it the necessary conditions for delivering services in a different manner that reflects the interests and views of those that use the service rather than those that provide it. The students appreciated the need to become more user focused and as suggested by Astedt-Kurki and Haggerman-Laitila (1992) only by 'identifying the criteria based on the clients own perception of services provided, will it ultimately be possible to penetrate the clients experiential world in greater depth and as a result respond appropriately to their needs'.

In summary, it is the concept of a 'therapeutic relationship' that still tends to dominate how students see their future role. Human qualities and attitudes were focused on; being approachable, showing respect and sensitivity, self awareness and understanding, a need to plan and structure listening time, informing, involving the family in promoting confidence and independence. The key knowledge base that was seen as desirable was about medication and talking therapies. However, there was much concern expressed as to the degree to which such care can be realised within practice. Clarke et al (1994 p203) indicate in the context of change that 'a key feature of the role of management is the stress it places on the "heroic" and "bold" role of senior managers in inspiring and enthusing workforces with a broader understanding of and commitment to the missions of the organisations for which they work'. It is hoped that the managerial (leadership) structure will be in place to enable the forthcoming generations of nurses to fulfil the role that they perceive for their future. It is also hoped that the student nurses will not ignore their individual responsibility in that role.

There was a considerable amount of convergence of how nurses and users perceive the role of the nurse and this is explored further in the next section.

TO WHAT EXTENT DO THE ANSWERS TO THE FIRST TWO QUESTIONS CONVERGE AND/OR DIVERGE?

Essentially, there was much convergence on issues relating to the need for genuine therapeutic relationships that focus precisely upon the needs of the individual and allow users to approach nurses for help on their terms rather than those of the system. There was agreement on the need for information to be much more freely available and for nurses to be at the forefront of providing information, which can help empower users and enable them to have greater control over treatment interventions and their lives generally. The desired principal role of the nurse was identified as social in orientation; that is, the nurse should engage with users not so much from a psychiatric diagnostic perspective but rather from one that focuses upon how users' mental distress affects their ability to function effectively in everyday life. Social skill training and social and economic factors were very much to the fore. Counselling and problem solving approaches were suggested, along with the ability to work with extended networks. There was convergence on the need for a mental health nurse to be older, that is, within their early thirties. It was believed that this could go some way in ensuring that nurses had some insight into problems of everyday living and the stress that can arise as a result. Students and users agreed that nurses had a responsibility to use research findings in order to develop their role on a much firmer foundation and act as agents of change. A significant convergence was the acknowledgement that users do not consistently experience in practice the desired interventions, support or appropriate attitudes.

There was some indecisive evidence from the data regarding the involvement of families and carers. There was a higher value attached to involving significant others by the nursing students than by the users, which we may conclude is due to the fact that users may not have a close-knit circle of friends and family and hence did not rate the issue so highly. This explanation would agree with the previously mentioned findings of Nolan and Clancy (1995) that indicated that despite users having attended rehabilitation programmes, many still led isolated and lonely lives in the community.

In response to the question relating to the nurse–user ratio, the students rated the issue as more important than the users but nevertheless not quite as convincingly as might have been expected. The general gist of the comments relating to this issue suggests that the users were more concerned about the quality of the nursing care, how nursing is organised and how nurses prioritise their work in terms of time spent with people or time on administrative duties. The students also drew attention to how qualified staff made use of their time but they did express concern over the number of staff available to enable nurses to do what they claim that they do. One comment suggested that the 'nurse–patient ratio is not satisfactory but even when it is, nurses tend to talk to each other in the office rather than with the patients'.

An issue that was raised in the Focus Groups but not ranked highly by the students was responding to the personal hygiene of users. The results from the questionnaire, although indecisive, tend to suggest that this is not a nurse's role and perhaps this is being seen as a role of the Health Care Assistant. However, for users it is through the personal interactions with the staff who provide the care that relationships are built and it is around such care that the importance of attitudes takes effect and qualities such as respect and compassion for the person can be demonstrated, or not.

Users wanted nurses to be more informed and aware about medical and physical conditions and rated this more highly than students. For users, this issue related to not being taken seriously which meant that real conditions were ignored and left untreated. Although students raised the issue in the Focus Groups and indicated that more knowledge about medical and physical conditions would be useful, it was not apparent that they shared the same perspective as users or were aware of the difficulty that users were experiencing in relation to the matter.

There was divergence in the responses relating to listening, with users indicating that nurses were not always prepared to listen to their views while the students suggested that they were. It may be that students answered this question on the basis of what they would do themselves, whereas users were reflecting their experience, which is consistent with evidence from the literature review. Campbell (1991) has suggested that 'the views of users are often not listened to, excluded and regarded as invalid simply on the grounds that they are users'. It may be that a stereotyped view of users continues to operate, which is that the 'mentally ill' cannot show any real insight and hence their ideas and opinions are disregarded. There will be times that users do not have any insight into their problems and they may express themselves inappropriately, but it does not follow that we should not listen to the views of users on the basis that they have a diagnosis of mental illness. The challenge is, can we make sense of what is being conveyed?

The use of physical restraint was highlighted as affecting the quality of user care but the results from the questionnaires were widespread and inconclusive as to whether users valued that role of the nurse. Some of the comments made by users suggested that physical restraint could be potentially a reassuring and protective intervention but that it was also one which users often experienced negatively as being an uncaring and an overpowering ordeal. Users saw managing aggression as part of the role of the nurse but expressed views that it needs to be done much more tactfully and sensitively. The students commented in the Focus Groups that physical restraint was part of the nurses' role and placed the issue in the context of managing aggression. Student discussion about physical restraint did not focus to any extent on its use in terms of a social control or a custodial role. It was not evident from their responses that they were aware of the issues that users were raising about the use of control and restraint, but that begs the question of whether there was an element of denial of the reality of physical restraint as used in practice.

Part of the nursing agenda that was at the forefront of the students' discussions, in positive terms, was the move to professional status. Students were keen that their improved education should lead to improved standing and saw the move in a wider context as a way of undermining traditional culture and power bases in mental health services, thereby improving the quality of care. Students expressed apprehension that they should be, and needed to be, confident and assertive if they were to be autonomous practitioners and act as agents of change. Although users shared the view that the traditional ways of delivering mental health services were not meeting their needs and that a fundamental shift in culture and control was required, from the responses and discussion of users about the nurses' role as professionals, some doubts and negativism were expressed. A shift of power from one professional body to another was clearly not part of the user agenda. Furthermore, in terms of their experience of the traditional hierarchies in practice, very often it was nurses who enacted the system of control.

Students' and users' perceptions are to a large extent convergent. This research shows that the students, having undergone the higher education preparation, did express a view of their role which reflected the concerns and expressed needs of users. However, although the correct utterances are being made they are not transformed into practice regularly or consistently. Users felt that lack of consistency is a key concern and that the quality of care depends on chance rather than on any systematic or conscious attempt to provide a high quality service. The preparation that students receive does not appear to be consistently enabling them to deliver in terms of users' needs once they are qualified. The evidence presented clearly suggests that a more humanistic, pluralistic and non-coercive system of support is required. In addressing the question of the role of the nurse, it appears clear that both users and the students place a high value on human caring qualities, the intangibles, and not any specialised behavioural, psychotherapy or psychoanalytical skills. These findings have an unequivocal implication for the education and training of mental health nurses and for further structural change.

RECOMMEND WAYS IN WHICH MENTAL HEALTH NURSING COULD BE IMPROVED, IN THE LIGHT OF THE FINDINGS OF THIS RESEARCH

Past reviews and inquiries into incidents within mental health services have resulted in many recommendations. The Mental Health Nursing Review of 1994 (Department of Health 1994) made 42 recommendations, *Learning the Lessons* (Zito & Howlett 1996) published by the Zito Trust listed 39 inquiries and over 300 recommendations, *Pulling Together* (Sainsbury Centre for Mental Health 1997) which looked at the future roles and training of mental health staff published in 1997 proposed a further 20. *Acute Problems* (Sainsbury Centre for Mental Health 1998) published in 1998, which investigated the quality of care in acute psychiatric wards recommended another 10. The National Service Framework (Department of Health 1999) for Mental Health, the *NHS Plan* (Department of Health 2000) and the reforming of the Mental Health Act and *Modernising the Care Programme Approach* (Department of Health 2001) all made further recommendations for change. Not all the recommendations relate to nursing, but nevertheless many have direct implications for nursing. So many recommendations dating back over ten years would suggest that we should now have a mental health service delivering outcomes of much higher quality than the experience of users indicates. Failure to achieve that high quality may give weight to the cynicism expressed by some users about the present service's ability to change. It may be that abundant recommendations result in important issues being lost and that those which might have led to really effective change from a user perspective are not being fed through to implementation. However, the remit of the Commission for Health Improvement (CHI) is to ensure that current policies are acted upon. The CHI is the independent authoritative voice on the state of the NHS in England and Wales and aims to improve the quality of patient care in the NHS by addressing unacceptable variations in NHS patient care, by identifying both notable practice and areas where care could be improved. CHI has six operating principles that underpin all of its work:

1. The patient's experience is at the heart of CHI's work.
2. CHI is independent, rigorous and fair.
3. CHI's approach is developmental and supports the NHS to continuously improve.
4. CHI's work is based on the best available evidence and focused on improvement.
5. CHI is open and accessible.
6. CHI applies the same standards of continuous improvement to itself that it expects of others and 'the patient's experience lies at the heart of CHI's work. We aim to improve standards by focusing on the experience of those using the NHS. We want the NHS to see itself as patients see it. Sometimes this process will be uncomfortable, but it is vital if the NHS is to provide a better service'. (Commission for Health Improvement 2004)

The following recommendations, based upon the findings from this research, may be placed within the context of two distinct broader options for the future of mental health nursing that will be discussed. It is intended that they are realistic and practicable to take forward in meeting the identified needs from a user and nursing perspective and helping to build appropriate opportunities for working in partnership to succeed.

KEY RECOMMENDATIONS

The key concerns that were identified and that require addressing are the following:

1. Users' views and opinions must be taken seriously with issues of real choices, participation, individuality and information giving being genuinely addressed.
2. Support must be provided in a compassionate and sensitive manner and nurses must be approachable and available for users.
3. Higher value should be placed on human caring qualities with appropriate attitudes and effective interpersonal skills, with genuine therapeutic relationships placed high on education and training agendas.
4. The gap in relation to users' social rehabilitation needs must be filled, with a focus placed upon social inclusion and the opportunity to acquire the necessary skills.
5. There should be continued development of a research base and the distinguishing of the best available evidence for practice.
6. There should be a reassessment of staffing levels, staff deployment and skill mix that recognises the need for administrative tasks and support.
7. The more senior, able and experienced staff should be the ones that spend the greater part of their time actually engaged with users in meeting their needs.
8. Rhetoric must be transformed into practice with a more humanistic, pluralistic and non-coercive system of support being developed.
9. Effective delivery of therapeutic intervention by those with the appropriate training and skills should be ensured.
10. We should continue to pursue a higher educated and skilled workforce in the context of defined outcomes for practice.
11. Recruitment and selection processes need examining and a recruitment policy considered which encourages applicants from an older and more experienced age group and from those who have had experience of being mental health service users.
12. There should be a greater focus upon how social needs, housing and employment relate to mental health.
13. The aim should be to effect real change in the structure and culture of the services as a whole, as at present it is not perceived as consistent or conducive to the promotion of therapeutic relationships that are user-centred.
14. The role ambiguity of nurses must be clarified if nursing is to be taken seriously as a profession with accountable and empowered nurses that are clear about their function within the context of user need and inter-professional working.

Option 1

From the findings it can be concluded that student nurses are in tune to a large extent with what users want from them. However, it may also be concluded from the views expressed by users that what they want is not being delivered in practice. Effective interpersonal skills and spending time with users should be a high priority but in practice this is not the case. The factors inhibiting the nurse–user relationship in practice have been previously discussed. Resource implications for having the time to talk have been considered, as have nurses' skill base in communicating, facilitating and effecting delivery of therapeutic intervention. Ritual task-orientated practice as a defence mechanism against anxiety in dealing with emotionally draining relationships, identified by Menzies (1970) over three decades ago, has also been considered as a continuing factor effecting the nurse–user relationship. These issues have been placed in the broader context of a service operating on an existing bedrock of culture, attitudes and established priorities; that is, a structure which resists the changes required to deliver a very different sort of service. Changes in education programmes have gone some way toward addressing some of the concerns that users wish to see addressed in preparing nurses to fulfil their role, but nurses are having difficulty in putting theory into practice. One argument is that the required cultural shift will not happen instantaneously and the changes in nurse education together with the structural changes within service delivery will produce the desired outcomes eventually. Only time will tell how effective the new generation of nurses are in delivering a more user-focused service. However, for the incrementalist approach to work further changes are needed in nursing education that address more fully the user agenda and there is a need to reassess, in terms of that agenda, the outcomes of some of the changes that have occurred.

The history of psychiatry and mental health show that those services have always been of a low priority and that staff were traditionally recruited from a pool of labour which was poorly educated, cheap to employ and ready to take orders (Hart 1994, Nolan 1993). Brooking (1985) also suggested that a poor level of education can lead to low standards of practice and refers to a 'vicious circle' of the continuing low level of care in mental health nursing: 1) Inadequate education; 2) Poorly educated nurses; 3) Lack of academic and research publications; 4) Practice based on ritual and routine rather than scientifically derived knowledge; 5) Poor quality patient care; 6) Low morale and loss of prestige; 7) Less well educated recruits attracted to nursing and 8) Lack of effective leaders and change agents. A better educated workforce may help to promote some of the desirable changes within the Health Service.

A general movement is underway in attempting to upgrade and professionalise nursing, having assessed that the benefit to patient care of more highly educated and trained nurses would be positive. But the changes that have taken place within health care services, deinstitutionalisation and greater emphasis towards the community, have meant that nurses have also gone through a period of role ambiguity and in many cases are still seeking their role identity. It is important that mental health nursing identifies not only key skills and core competencies but also the appropriate aptitudes and attitudes necessary for effective and qualitative delivery of services that are firmly based on the needs of their client group. If an increased knowledge of users' perspectives does not lead to relevant interventions then what is the purpose of such knowledge other than as an exercise in intellectual gymnastics or the promotion and defence of professions?

This research has identified various outcomes that users perceive as being pertinent to their needs. The notion of a therapeutic relationship has long been an issue of attention and again this is identified as a key component. The extent to which nurses in practice engage in such relationships and thereby make an impact on outcomes remains questionable. Although many users have been able to identify certain individuals who have engaged with them in a genuine endeavour to meet their needs, the structure and culture of the services as a whole are not perceived as consistent or conducive to the promotion of therapeutic relationships that are fundamentally user centred. Mental health nursing must move away from the rhetoric of therapeutic relationships and act on the best available evidence to transform the rhetoric into reality. Nurses must do what they say they do and be accountable for quality interventions. In this changing climate of health care provision it has become increasingly important for nursing to show that the input nurses give has a clear output to the user of the service. They need to be able to identify and separate the factors that lead to distress, be they organic, social, psychological or political, and respond accordingly to the identified need.

It is essentially through an interpersonal relationship that an understanding of an individual can be achieved, but the indications are that many of the senior clinical nursing staff spend much of their time on administrative duties that keep them away from service users. The building of effective relationships, which has been recognised as high on the agenda throughout the period researched, and is acknowledged as the core skill for mental health nurses, is more often left to untrained colleagues. Refering again to the findings of Gijbels (1995) study, in practice, therapeutic nursing activities were given lower priority by qualified nurses than other activities. Mental health nurses must have the skills to engage effectively if they are to work in partnership with users and they must also be prepared to be in the front line using those skills. It appears that there is a need to reassess the skill mix that operates in care-giving environments and to ask whether nurses need to be doing some of the administrative and organisational tasks that take them away from users when other personnel could be employed to do these things. It is important to acknowledge the issues uncovered by Menzies (1970) in the 1960s and to acknowledge that these are continuously relevant to nursing practice, and ask what coping mechanisms nurses are using to deal with emotionally draining interaction and to what extent these are being ritualised as an accepted part of the structure. Nurse training needs to focus on the realities of having to deliver within the emotional environment that is the setting for mental health services. Nurses must be made fully aware of the demands that they will be expected to cope with and helped to develop coping mechanisms that are not detrimental to user care. It cannot be expected that recently qualified nurses can cope effectively in practice without a solid structure of support, which should involve clinical supervision.

The use of health care assistants has been an attempt to introduce a skill mix within nursing practice with the assistants doing the so-called basic tasks requiring lower skills levels and consequently receiving lower pay. However, it is questionable whether there has been a proper definition of these basic tasks in the case of mental health nursing care. Health care assistants are actually performing front line tasks but without appropriate education and training whilst the nurses do, to all intents and purposes, administrative tasks. Carr-Hill et al (1992) have warned that the introduction of health care assistants with very little training could undermine the progressive changes towards a more professional ethos within nursing. Walby and Greenwell (1994) also suggest that these developments could lead to a polarisation between the higher trained and qualified diploma and degree level nurse and an increasingly dense layer of numerous health care assistants. Nurses are also increasingly working agency, bank or part time and such temporary nurses are unlikely to develop an ongoing knowledge of the ward, unit or users, detracting from the attempt by nursing leaders to upgrade the whole profession. Users want to be cared for by nurses who consider nursing as a career, which users see as reflecting the right attitude and commitment. There is a danger that the system is yet again setting the wrong priorities in practice and service managers need to think carefully about the priority expectations they are projecting.

The ability to engage therapeutically with users involves rather intangible qualities and the degree to which these can be taught is debatable. In this research the students put a high value on education but users put a greater value on 'caring qualities'. Nursing and therapy are about being with and trying to understand people's experiences and this poses a challenge to those responsible for the education and the preparation of nurses. For example, how can the development of empathy and personal insight be measured? During the 1980s and 1990s nursing has become preoccupied with becoming a profession, and the need to create a specific body of nursing knowledge. Research to establish such a body of knowledge has been pursued vigorously since the closure of traditional Schools of Nursing and the transfer of nurse education into the university sector (although it is highly debatably whether nurse education has really integrated into higher education). Many nurse education centres have remained on NHS locations, are somewhat apart from other disciplines and do not have the same academic year. Acquiring knowledge is a different process than developing the 'self' and it is the development of the 'self' in terms of the intangible caring qualities that is highly valued by users and needs to be given a much higher profile. An individual develops and changes attitudes through life experiences, so is it really possible for a structured education process to address this issue? This type of learning cannot be delivered in the traditional academic format but is a process of experiential learning and this must also be offered within colleges and universities.

However, there are difficulties with this. The unprecedented rate of change that has taken place within nursing and its move into higher education has meant that in many cases, larger group sizes tend to prevail. This mitigates against effective experiential teaching that could be used to explore the issues of self awareness within smaller groups and within psychologically safe environments. Large seminar groups or lecture formats do not lend themselves to any real exploration of the individual. Research carried out by Gibbs (1996) indicates that students dislike large class sizes and adopt a surface approach to learning, achieve lower marks and to a greater extent operate at lower cognitive levels. The large group culture could negate some of the more positive aspects of the move into universities since what users are asking for may not be effectively developed within large groups or lecture theatres. Nurse preparation as a developmental process for the individual student would require a greater emphasis on experiential learning in facilitated groups that also has implications for the skills of the nurse teacher/lecturer. According to Turunen et al (1997) the move to universities has been a way of breaking with the past where the style of teaching in traditional nurse education settings tended to encourage dependence rather than autonomy in nurses. However, it must be borne in mind that the academic who can deliver effective lectures to large groups may not have the skills to facilitate personal development within smaller groups. It is also questionable whether there has been a significant cultural change away from a dependency culture to an autonomous one.

The 1968 review emphasised the separate training and identity of the Registered Mental Nurse (RMN). Equally, the 1994 review continued to support the notion of specialist qualification at initial pre-registration level and that mental health nursing should not become a post-registration speciality. It can be argued that mental health nursing should be kept separate and distinct from general nursing to encourage a move away from the medical model that being tied to general nursing tends to imply. The current pre-registration syllabus of training comprises a one-year common foundation and two-year branch programme leading to a diploma or a degree, although the common foundation programme continues to have more of a general nursing culture and agenda. The idea of all nurse preparation being at degree level with a generic qualification is also still on the agenda and is seen by some as a way forward for nursing. Gournay (1996) argues that the notion of the generic nurse is a development that would contribute to the demise of the mental health nurse. It is quite clear that the reforms of nurse education have not fully addressed the training requirements of mental health nursing, as a two-year branch preparation is not sufficient time for developing the skills, knowledge and attitudes that the findings of this research suggest are necessary.

There is a move in many areas of employment that involves working with vulnerable client groups to look at staff in relation to their overall fitness to do the job. Employers have expressed concern that individuals may present with qualifications, although these do not indicate whether they have the appropriate personality or attitude. Specific skills training is easier if the individual has the appropriate attitude; skills can be acquired more easily on the job if the commitment is there to do so. The 1994 review focused on the skills that nurses are required to have and produced an extensive list, but it is dubious whether this actually helps to identify what a nurse who is fit for purpose should be like. There is a need to consider a 'fit person' definition in relation to mental health nursing that is not just a long list of skills which may be utilised as a checklist of topics to include in the nurse-training syllabus, but that ensures there is a commitment to enter into career-long learning and attempts to define an appropriate attitude. It must be acknowledged that there is not the time in pre-registration to cover the wide range of knowledge and skills that nurses will find they need to draw upon in their career, but time must be found to cover what is important and to ensure that the newly qualified nurse is a 'fit-person' for the role.

If there is a limit to the extent that commitment and attitude can be taught then we must look more critically at the mechanisms being used by colleges and universities to define aptitude at the point of selection, and at the selection process generally. However, the contract culture poses problems for a quality selection process. Universities are endeavouring to achieve contracted numbers of students for Trusts before the commencement of courses, which places an emphasis on quantity rather than quality. Once students start a course there needs to be a means of exiting students early who are deemed unsuitable because of their aptitude and attitude. Unfortunately, this can be rather difficult since contracts for the education and training of nurses tend to include claw back clauses of funds if target numbers are not achieved. This situation can lead to much undesirable compromise in terms of the calibre of students recruited, and reluctance to discontinue unsuitable candidates. The shortage of nurses and the Government's drive to recruit more nursing students will intensify this process.

The findings presented in this book have confirmed that users needs in terms of social and economic integration and the problems associated with stigma are fundamental, widespread and are not being sufficiently addressed. Users felt that nurses had a major role in addressing these unmet needs and that the mental health agenda must ensure that users are understood and helped within the context of their immediate social and economic system and within a wider view of their world, as people do not and cannot live in vacuums. There needs to be a changed perception of mental illness that invites different forms of interventions and help of which medical professionals have no claim to expertise, for example housing, employment, social and leisure activities. Users are no longer seeing work as part of therapy per se but as an essential move away from the culture of dependency and towards economic and social integration. There is no doubt that practical solutions must be considered in order to begin to address these fundamental problems and if the aim of community care and the improvement of the social functioning of those with mental health problems is to be realised, then nurses need to familiarise themselves with current research into user views. They must effectively assess what users' health and social needs are, specifically, and what kind of assistance is required, and be instrumental in initiating the necessary support. Nurses are potentially in an effective position to provide practical support to users, to foster real partnership and take up their cause and to help address the real consequences of social stigma.

Users are clearly telling us that the medical model of psychiatry is not addressing their concerns. The science of neurology is important for furthering our understanding about ourselves and of course medication can have positive and helpful effects in alleviating distress. However, that does not justify basing the whole structure of care services for those with mental health problems around that science. Users are saying they want help in different ways and there is an opportunity for nurses to deliver in those ways. There is much potential within mental health nursing practice but often it withers away and is lost. Nurses who genuinely wish to meet the needs of users must become more politically conscious and be proactive in responding to the agenda of the day with a clear vision of what is required in providing a qualitative user-focused service.

The findings of this research suggest that if nurses are to be trained in a way that enables them to respond to a mental health user agenda then curriculum development must focus on the following areas:

1. Improvement of self-awareness, assess attitudes and prejudices and ensure that nurses become aware of the emotional demands that their role will entail and their recourse to coping strategies.
2. Develop interpersonal skills.
3. Impart skills to facilitate groups effectively within the context of an individual's care plan.
4. Teach a collaborative approach to care in assessing users' needs with working in partnership as a key focus.
5. Develop counselling skills and skills to conduct effective talking therapy.
6. A greater emphasis on the social and economic context of users' lives and setting this within the therapeutic framework.
7. Provide training in relation to effective rehabilitation, which focuses on the social and economic reintegration needs of users, which would include issues around equal opportunities and the effects of stereotypes within society.
8. More intense and facilitated discussion around issues of integrity and professionalism and, within this context, an examination of issues of power and politics within systems, and particularly, within mental health services and how change is effected. Make links to how smaller teams and individuals operate within systems and how they in particular will function in performing their role in practice. The aim is

to enable nurses to maintain their integrity in fulfilling the role for which they have been prepared.

Option 2

The structure and culture of mental health services at all levels need challenging if nursing is to become unshackled from its conservative chains of tradition. Hopton (1997) argues that despite the self-image of mental health nursing by many as innovative, radical and progressive, he perceives this as 'false consciousness' and suggests that, 'Mental health nursing can never develop truly liberating approaches to care unless it widens its focus from purely interpersonal approaches and addresses historical, structural and ideological influences on both mental health services and the causation of mental distress'.

The findings in this research do give credence for a more pessimistic view of whether the service in which the mental health nurse has a central role, but still within the medical/psychiatric structure of accountability and control, can ever deliver the sort of service that users want. The implication is that a new agenda in nurse education will not deliver the required changes in the service without structural changes in the way that mental health services are being run which go to the heart of control and accountability. Arguments within this book have suggested that the changes occurring in the service, most dramatically the move to community care, are not going far enough. Many student nurses expressed their concerns that enthusiastic newly qualified nurses are quickly being assimilated into existing practice culture that tends to negate some of the positive changes that could occur. If mental health nurses are not able to move away from their historical chains that tend to anchor them to inertia then perhaps the time has come to welcome the demise of mental health nursing and to create in its wake a health care worker that is genuinely responsive and effective in meeting the needs of those who need a mental health service. If nurses allow complacency to prevail rather than being proactive then nurses should not be surprised when the abolition of mental health nursing is advocated.

We have already seen the introduction of the Graduate Mental Health Worker that may be a welcomed thin end of a wedge. They represent a new breed of mental health worker whose introduction departs from the usual routes into mental health work. It is anticipated that they will be graduates who have a first degree in social science or psychology and undertake a one-year work-based course that has been devised with health care trusts, users and carers and will lead to a postgraduate certificate in primary care mental health practice. On successful completion of the programme, they will continue to work in their Primary Care Trust. *The NHS Plan* recognised that primary care needed resources to build additional capacity and set a target of 1, 000 Primary Care Graduate Mental Health Workers to be in post in by December 2004. These workers constitute a new kind of mental health worker who will be trained specifically to improve access to mental health support in primary care in order to help meet the *NHS Plan* and National Service Framework requirements for mental health. They will be trained to deliver three main roles:

- face to face work with clients with common mental health problems such as anxiety and depression;
- work within the practice team including liaising with service users and carers, practise audit and activities such as the setting up and management of mental illness case registers;
- networking with the wider health and social care system.

This new intake of workers may be the beginning of substantive changes in mental health services and could make a big difference in perhaps helping to change the current culture. However, there will also be those who will oppose such developments and endeavour to denigrate such changes. Some user groups are also moving in the direction of setting up their own services and Hopton and Glenister (1996) point out that the Arbours Association has successfully provided independent health care for over twenty-five years without employing nurses as such, preferring to induct all staff and helpers through their own training scheme. Thus an option would be to acknowledge that the current situation is beyond reform and that State provision should be set up as a new service to deliver on a new agenda.

This book has considered how stereotypes reflect and have real implications for the way people are treated and how they treat others and has acknowledged the importance of semantics in reinforcing stereotypes. The stereotype of the mentally ill patient is mirrored in society by the psychiatric/mental health nurse who is perceived as being in the business of custodial care, operating within a control structure run by psychiatrists. Users are clear that they do not want to be the stereotyped patient, and student nurses are clear that they do not want to be the stereotyped nurse. A new title for those delivering mental health care could be the first step to the reality of a new breed of mental health worker delivering a new service that is not under the umbrella of psychiatry or operating within a medical model. The Consultant Psychiatrist, with clinical responsibility in law, would no longer be in charge. New structures of responsibility, accountability and control could be set up at the heart of the service and other specialised professional input could be drawn on as required. A new structure could build upon new definitions of service delivery and outcomes and provide the opportunity for users to become more involved and have greater influence. Such a scenario could allow a fundamental redefining of the required skill base and skill mix of those working in the service and provide a real opportunity for professional status and research. A professional mental health worker may present an attractive career option for a broader section of the population and encourage applicants who would not have chosen to be nurses.

The new breed of mental health worker that is perhaps a combination of a mental health nurse, a psychologist and a social worker could help to integrate social and health care needs. A challenge for mental health services is the growing need for a better integration of health and social services as this separation has often resulted in poor communication and problems that could be avoided as a result of one sector making decisions without consulting the other. The review team responsible for the *Working in Partnership Report* (Department of Health 1994 p9) were ready 'to consider the creation of a new type of mental health care worker, but received little evidence to support such a development'. Perhaps the research that has been undertaken into the views of service users since the review will add to the evidence required that suggests that such a venture is now not only desirable but also possible. Whether there is the political will for such structural change is debatable given the inevitable resource implications and great infringement of vested interests and power bases. There would be formidable difficulties in dismantling a service that has been in existence for many years, regardless of its relative ineffectiveness. However, developments within the European community may lend impetus to the demise of the mental health nurse given that Britain, Ireland and the Netherlands are the only countries that have pre-registration mental health nursing education and training. There has been a European Directive since 1979 recognising general nursing qualifications and the mobility of labour between member states, but with no directive for mental health nursing.

A report produced by a Project Team from the University of Manchester (1996) entitled *The Future Healthcare Workforce* set out to answer the question, 'If we were designing the workforce today for tomorrow's Health Service, what would it look like?' In reply to the question it is suggested that there is a need to tackle both the supply and demand side of the labour force equation. Part of the solution they proposed was to transfer a significant proportion of the workload to other non-professional personnel. They cite evidence from industry that shows that the ability to switch staff between different tasks can be extremely valuable to workplace efficiency. The merging of roles and the changing boundaries of responsibilities would help create a more flexible workforce, give employees more autonomy on job design which in turn could reflect local need and appropriate services. In essence, a generic carer would be responsible for the co-ordination of the service and the majority of user care. Education and training would be to produce a generic worker who is more clearly focused on the requirements of the job rather than single occupational professionals. The report further suggests that by the year 2005 the 'generic carer' will constitute 40% of the workforce. The report *Pulling Together* published by the Sainsbury Centre for Mental Health (1997) identified a need for a complete review of education and training of all mental health professionals. It highlighted the need for more effective training in meeting the requirements of users and carers and found skills deficits in the area of rehabilitation. It suggests that core competencies for mental health workers need to be established across all specialities and a core curriculum introduced. It upholds that all staff require much better training in effective team and partnership working and that some kind of joint education and training is essential to enhance mental health services.

There has been much change during the last decade and it is likely that changes will continue during the next ten years. It remains to be seen whether nursing has the determination and the maturity to respond to this challenge, or whether it will proceed as described by Fabricius (1991) as 'running on the spot'. Running on the spot she regards as a certain manic tendency within nursing to change things without grappling with the fundamental problems. She defines the concept as 'an outwardly major change that may shift the dynamics a little, before they settle down into the same state of equilibrium that existed before, even if it is maintained in a slightly different way'.

As Machiavelli (1961) proclaimed, 'it should be borne in mind that there is nothing more difficult to handle, more doubtful of success, and more dangerous to carry through than initiating change'. The problem may be that if mental health nurses do not grasp the nettle of change, it may proceed without them.

References

Alden L 1978 Treatment environment and patient improvement. Journal of Nervous and Mental Disease 166(5):327-334

Astedt-Kurki P, Haggman-Laitila A 1992 Good practices as perceived by clients: a starting point for the development of professional nursing. Journal of Advanced Nursing 17:1195-1199

Bergin A E, Soloman S 1994 Personality and performance correlates of empathic understanding in psychotherapy. In: Rolfe G (ed) Some factors associated with change in patient-centredness of student nurses during the common foundation programme in nursing. International Journal of Nursing Studies 31(5):422

Blom-Cooper L, Hally H, Murphy E 1995 The falling shadow. Duckworth, London

Brooking J 1985 Advanced psychiatric nurse training in Britain. Journal of Advanced Nursing 10:455-468

Butterworth T, Faugier J 1992 Clinical supervision and mentoring in nursing. Chapman and Hall, London

Campbell P 1991 From the video - we're not mad, we're angry. Mental Health Media, London

Campbell P 1996 Working with service users. In: Sandford T, Gournay K (eds) Perspectives in mental health nursing. Bailliere Tindall, London

Carkhuff R R, Kratochvil D, Friel T 1968 The effects of graduate training. Journal of Couselling Psychology 15:68-74

Carr-Hill R, Higgins M, DixonP et al 1992 Skill mix and the effectiveness of nursing care: a report to the Department of Health. Centre for Health Economics, University of York

Clarke C, Cochrane A, McLaughlin E 1994 Managing social policy. Sage, London

Commission for Health Improvement 2004 Online. Available: http:/ /www.chi.gov.ik/eng/about/whatischi.shtml#00

Department of Health 1994 Working in partnership - report of the Mental Health Nursing Review Team. HMSO, London

Department of Health 1994 Working in partnership - report of the Mental Health Nursing Review Team. HMSO, London

Department of Health 1999 National services framework for mental health. Stationary Office, London

Department of Health 2000 The NHS plan. Stationary Office, London

Department of Health 2001 Modernising the care programme approach. Stationary Office, London

Dooley F 1999 The named nurse in practice. Nursing Standard 13(34):33-38

Egan G 1998 The skilled helper. Brooks Cole, California

Fabricius J 1991 Running on the spot or can nursing really change? Psychoanalytical Psychotherapy 15(2):97-108

Farley A, Hendry C 1992 Critical and constructive. Nursing Times 88(39):36

Georgiades N J, Phillimore L 1975 The myth of the hero innovator. In: Kiernan C C, Woodford F P (eds) Behaviour modification with the severely retarded. Associated Scientific, London

Gibbs G 1996 Using research to improve student learning in large classes. Oxford Centre for Staff Development, Oxford

Gijbel H 1995 Mental health nursing skills in an acute admission environment: perceptions of mental health nurses and other health care professionals. Journal of Advanced Nursing 21:462

Gijbels H, Burnard P 1995 Exploring the skills of mental health nurses. Avebury, Aldershot

Gournay K 1996 Changes and challenges - the future of mental health nursing. In: Sandford T, Gournay K (eds) Perspectives in mental health nursing. Bailliere Tindall, London

Hall J A, Dornan M C 1988 What patients like about their medical care and how often they are asked : a meta analysis of the satisfaction literature. Social Science and Medicine 27:935-939

Hart C 1994 Behind the mask. Bailliere Tindall, London

Hogg C 1994 Beyond the patients charter: working with users. Health Rights. London

Hopton J 1997 Towards a critical theory of mental health nursing. Journal of Advanced Nursing 25:492

Hopton J, Glenister D 1996 Working in partnership: vision or pipe dream? Journal of Theory and Practice in Social Welfare 47:111-119

Jackson S, Stevenson C 1998 The gift of time from the friendly professional. Nursing Standard 12(5):31-33

Kammerling R, O'Connor S 1993 Unemployment rate as a predictor of rate of psychiatric admission. British Medical Journal 307:1536-1539

Lovell K 1995 User satisfaction with in-patient mental health services. Journal of Psychiatric and Mental Health Nursing 2(3):143-150

Machiavelli N 1961 The prince. (translated by Bull G.) Penguin, Harmondsworth

Martin J P 1984 Hospitals in trouble. Blackwell, London

Masson J 1988 Against therapy. Harper-Collins, New York

McGonagle I M, Gentle J 1996 Reasons for non-attendance at a day hospital for people with enduring mental illness: the clients perspective. Journal of Psychiatric and Mental Health Nursing 3(1):61-66

Meltzer H, Gill B, Petticrew M, Hinds K 1995 Economic activity and social functioning of adults with psychiatric disorders. Office of Population Censuses and Surveys. HMSO, London

Mental Health Act Commission/The Sainsbury Centre for Mental Health 1997 The national visit. The Sainsbury Centre for Mental Health, London

Mental Health Foundation 1997 Knowing our own minds: a survey of how people in emotional distress take control of their lives. Mental Health Foundation, London

Menzies I 1970 Social systems as a defence against anxiety. Reprinted as Tavistock pamphlet no. 3. Tavistock Institute of Human Relations, London

National Health Service Executive 1995 Code of practice on openness in the NHS. NHS Executive, Leeds

Nolan P 1990 Psychiatric nursing - the first 100 years. Senior Nurse 10(10):20-23

Nolan P 1993 A history of mental health nursing. Chapman and Hall, London

Nolan P, Clancy A 1995 A survey of social networks of people with severe mental health problems. Journal of Psychiatric and Mental Health Nursing 2(3):131-142

Prail T, Baldwin S 1988 Beyond hero-innovation: real changes in unreal systems. Behaviour Psychotherapy 16:1-14

Rogers A, Pilgrim D, Lacey R 1993 Experiencing psychiatry. Macmillan/MIND, Basingstoke

Rogers C 1951 Client centered therapy. Houghton Mufflin, Boston

Rolfe G 1990 The assessment of therapeutic attitudes in the psychiatric setting. Journal of Advanced Nursing 21:564-570

Rose D 1996 Living in the community. The Sainsbury Centre for Mental Health, London

Sainsbury Centre for Mental Health 1997 Pulling together. The Sainsbury Centre for Mental Health, London

Sainsbury Centre for Mental Health 1998 Acute problems. The Sainsbury Centre for Mental Health, London

Sheldon K 1997 When the tables turn. Nursing Times 93(11):34-36

Sundeen S, Stuart G, Rankin E, Cohen S 1985 Nurse-client interaction. Mosby, Missouri

Turunen H, Taskinen H, Voutilainen U et al 1997 Nursing ans social work students initial orientation towards their studies. Nurse Education Today 17:67-71

University of Manchester 1996 The future healthcare workforce: the steering group report commissioned by the National Association of Health Authorities and Trusts. University of Manchester, Manchester

University of Manchester 1996 The future healthcare workforce: the steering group report. Commissioned by the National Association of Health Authorities and Trusts. Manchester University, Manchester

Van Ooijen E 1994 Whipping up a storm. Nursing Standard 9(8):48

Walby S, Greenwell J 1994 Managing the National Health Service. In: Clarke J, Cochrane A, McLaughlin E (eds) Managing social policy. Sage, London

Weldon F 1997 Mind at the end of its tether. The Guardian 11 January

Wright H 1989 Group work: perspectives and practice. Scutari, London

Zito J, Hpwlett M 1996 Introduction. In: Sheppard D (ed) Learning the lessons. The Zito Trust, London

Chapter 8

Conclusion

INTRODUCTION

The aim of this book was to examine the notion of partnership in care and to evaluate the role of mental health nursing in achieving partnership working and in meeting the needs of users of mental health services; to report on the research findings of how users perceive their needs and the degree to which they are being met; and to ascertain what changes are required in the preparation and the role of the mental health nurse as a key player in users' care in a service where users' needs are not being met. It is hoped the book will promote a greater understanding of those issues, as it is vital for professionals in mental health services to be fully aware of the real outcomes of their work if they are to move forward in making working in partnership a reality. The latter part of the 20th century has seen much criticism of mental health services. Mono causal medical explanations of mental illness were no longer acceptable to many users who were beginning to find their voice and to challenge the bastions of power and the established knowledge base. With a greater focus on community care, users are demanding different treatment other than drugs to meet their needs and users want their needs to be defined in the context of everyday living. The dissatisfaction with mental health services has given rise to a user movement that has gone from strength to strength. Many mental health policy documents speak about the need to hear the real voice of service users, which has made an impact upon policy direction with users being involved in many decision-making bodies.

Mental health services in England are experiencing a period of exceptional challenge and change. The Government (Department of Health 2004) suggests that,

> 'only the pace at which information about both effective and less effective practice in mental health care is emerging potentially matches the pace of this change. Over the past five years an incredible wealth of published literature has continued to remind all those engaged in developing mental health services of the reasons why fundamental change is necessary and of how services might be improved to better meet the needs of service users'.

Thus, at the turn of the millennium the issues of user perspective hasg been firmly placed on the mental health agenda. We have seen an increase in user-focused literature and a genuine move towards the notion of users as partners in care, although not all published literature will find its way to those professionals who are best placed to act on the evidence. There will be some professionals who are not proactive or, worse, not interested in keeping up with research, literature and policy as a basis for achieving best practice. Others may argue that there is limited space in their intensely busy working lives to do so. Thus the dissemination of research findings and official policies often takes time to catch up with the relevant audiences. Despite the abundance of research, stated policy intentions and increased user involvement, change at every day practice level is slow.

There have been some positive changes over the past decade. We have witnessed the closure of the large Victorian institutions that primarily saw the work of the nurse as ensuring cleanliness, maintaining order and carrying out medical orders. The emphasis on routine and task-led care has diminished and nurses are endeavouring, at least in theory, to devote more energy and time to the human needs of patients, but there is a long way to go. There is still a need to move away from a custodial approach to care and towards a more therapeutic relationship with more meaningful activities and involvement with users. Communication skills, psychology and sociology were introduced into all basic nurse training courses as an attempt to broaden an understanding of mental distress and to appreciate the context of users' lives. We have also seen the consolidation of the need to focus upon nurses' relationships with users and for nursing to develop as a profession and to assert its integrity in the face of institutional pressures to conform. Current nursing literature and research continues to reflect the commitment to the quality of interpersonal relations in the work of the nurse. The findings presented here are in agreement with the importance placed upon the intangible qualities that are at the heart of interpersonal relationships and the need to further develop these within nursing. However, the data presented in this book shows that users do not always feel that their perspectives on their distress are taken seriously enough and that they are still mainly engaged with as an illness label rather than as fellow human beings with basic human needs. The notion of a meaningful 'therapeutic relationship', which mental health nursing proclaims as its quintessence, is what users are asking for but it is not regularly or consistently experienced in practice; the standards and quality of care identified as desirable are not being met. Nevertheless, this research shows that there is much convergence on the views of users and nurses on what is important and what needs to be changed. It is reasonable to conclude that at a theoretical level, much of what is being taught about the concept of nursing and the role of the nurse is appropriate in that it converges with the views of users.

The change in nurse preparation hopes to produce nurses that are flexible, knowledgeable and free thinkers. The purpose of their education is to build confidence and self esteem as well as imparting knowledge. This research shows that the participating student nurses felt that they were receiving education to fit those criteria. Their concerns reflected their future within practice. The research suggests that they saw from their clinical placements that nurses still spend a great deal of their time on administrative work rather than engaging in effective interpersonal relationships and working in partnership with users. They had doubts that the aspiration to achieve a quality service remained a priority for the qualified nurse in practice or that the qualified nurse pursued the aim with any persistence or determination. They feared that the culture within mental health nursing would erode their self-confidence. It is difficult to conclude that nurses can build a real sense of self worth or feel that they are fulfilling a professional role if their time is being spent on administrative work. If, however, they are seeking emotional refuge in administrative work, that may lead to the question of whether education is actually imparting the necessary interpersonal skills and sustaining such skills in practice.

The research was undertaken in an endeavour to attain an understanding of the participants' point of view of their experiences. The reliability of the research is important if it is to be useful in informing practise. Unless we listen properly to the views of those who use the services, working in partnership will never be achieved. Throughout this research an attempt was made to avoid data misrepresentation, as the aim was to achieve an end result that was an accurate reflection of user and nursing issues. The participants raised the issue of misrepresentation on a few occasions; both users and students were concerned about the possibility of having their views distorted. The many quotes within this book are the verbatim words of the research participants and have been presented in a manner and context that is true to their position. The research does carry issues of representation. As the groups were self-selecting in agreeing to participate in the research, there was no control over whether they had a particular grievance and were keen to speak out against the system. Therefore, it needs to be borne in mind that the research cannot claim that participants and their views are representative of all mental health service user groups or all mental health nursing students.

It is hoped that some of the issues identified will be followed up. Areas for further review that have come to light from the data are:

- The need to look at examples of user-run services, to establish how they are operating and how effective they are;
- To check the experiences of newly qualified nurses;
- To explore the views of senior nurse managers about their perception of the role of the mental health nurse;
- To monitor the degree to which the social and economic needs of users are being addressed.

The research has confirmed that, above all, there must be a permanent change in the balance of power between those who use mental health services and those who provide services if a genuine, quality, mental health care service is to prevail. Listening and responding to the needs of those who use services is an important part of making change effective and achieving genuine partnership working. The National Institute for Mental Health in England (NIMHE) (2004) that was set up in June 2002 states as its mission statement:

'We aim to improve the quality of life for people of all ages who experience mental distress. Working beyond the NHS, we help all those involved in mental health to implement positive change, providing a gateway to learning and development, offering new opportunities to share experiences and one place to find information. Through NIMHE's local development centres and national programmes of work, we will support staff to put policy into practice and to resolve local challenges in developing mental health. To achieve these aims, service users, families and communities will be at the heart of our work. We will embrace diversity, champion achievements, help to break down bureaucracy and promote flexible ways of working. NIMHE is forging new partnerships at a national and international level. We will take a lead in connecting mental health research, development, delivery, monitoring and review.'

We need to make sure that all professionals working within mental health services not only subscribe to that statement of intent but also act it out in practice.

References

Department of Health 2004 Online. Available: http://www.doh.gov.uk/mentalhealth

National Institute for Mental Health in England 2004 Online. Available: http://www.nimhe.org.uk/about/index.asp

Appendix

Bibliography

Audit Commission 1994 Finding a place - a review of mental health services for adults. HMSO, London

Barker P 1996 Chaos and the way of Zen. Journal of Psychiatric and Mental Health Nursing 3(4):235-243

Barker P 2003 Psychiatric and mental health nursing. Arnold, London

Barton W R 1959 Institutional neurosis. Wright, Bristol

Beeforth M, Conlan E, Graley R 1994 Have we got views for you: users evaluation of case management. The Sainsbury Centre for Mental Health, London

Behi R, Nolan M 1995 Ethical issues in research. British Journal of Nursing 4(12):712-716

Beresford P 2000 Our voice in our future. Mental health issues. National Institute for Social Work, London

Better Regulation Task Force 1999 Fit person criteria. Central Office for Information, London

Black J 1992 User involvement in mental health services: an annotated bibliography 1985-1992. Department of Social Policy and Social Work, Birmingham University

Brandon D 1991 Innovations without change? Consumer power in psychiatric services. Macmillan, London

Brealey S 1990 Patient participation: the literature. Scutari, Harrow

Burnard P 1995 Unspoken meanings: qualitative research and multi-media analysis. Nurse Researcher 3(1):55-64

Butler T 1993 Changing mental health services - the politics and policy. Chapman and Hall, London

Butterworth T 1994 Developing research ideas from theory into practice: psychosocial interventions as a case example. Nurse Researcher 1(4):78-86

Butterworth T 1995 The current status and future challenges of psychiatric/mental nursing. Internatinal Journal of Nursing Studies 32(4):353-365

Campbell P, Lindow V 1997 Changing practice: mental health nursing and user empowerment. MIND/RCN, London

Cavanagh S 1997 Content analysis: concepts, methods and applications. Nurse Researcher 4(3):5-15

Chan P 1998 Paternalistic intervention in mental health care. Nursing Times 94(36):52-53

Clutterbuck D 1995 The power of empowerment. Kogan Page, London

Crawford P, Brown B, Nolan P 1998 Communicating care. Stanley Thornes, Cheltenham

Department of Health 1998 Our healthier nation. HMSO, London

Department of Health 2001 The journey to recovery - the Government's vision for mental health care. Department of Health, London

English National Board for Nursing, Midwifery and Health Visiting 1996 Learning from each other: the involvement of people who use services and their carers in education and training. ENB, London

Erickson B H, Nosanchuk T A 1993 Understanding data. Open University, Buckingham

Faulkner A 1997 Knowing our own minds: a survey of how people in emotional distress take control of their lives. Mental Health Foundation, London

Fukuyama F 1999 The great disruption. Profile Books, London

Gabe J, Kelleher D, Williams G 1994 Challenging medicine. Routledge, London

Glenister D 1994 Patient participation in psychiatric services: a review and proposal for a research strategy. Journal of Advanced Nursing 19:802-811

Gordon C 1986 Psychiatry as a problem of democracy. In: Millar P, Rose N (eds) The power of psychiatry. Polity, Cambridge

Hamilton S, Farebrother S 1995 Involving users in a review of mental health service provision. Mental Health Nursing 15(4):12-14

Harrison S, Hunter D, Marnoch G, Pollitt C 1992 Just managing: power and culture in the NHS. Macmillan, London

Health Committee 1994 First report - better off in the community? - The care of people who are seriously mentally ill, Vol 1. HMSO, London

Hickey G, Kipping C 1998 Who becomes a mental nurse? Nursing Times 94(31):53-54

Hill B, Michael S 1996 The human factor. Journal of

Psychiatric and Mental Nursing 3(4):245-248

Hopton J 1995 The application of the idea of Franze Fanon to the practice of mental health nursing. Journal of Advanced Nursing 21:723-728

Krueger R A 1994 Focus groups: a practical guide for applied research. Sage, London

Lindow V 1994 Self help alternatives to mental health services. MIND, London

Lukes S 1974 Power: a radical view. Macmillan, London

McIver S 1991 Obtaining the view of users of health services. MIND, London

Merton R K, Kendall P L 1946 The focused interview. American Journal of Sociology 51(6):541-557

Ministry of Health 1961 Short stay psychiatric unit. Hospital building not no. 5. HMSO, London

Morse J 1997 Completing a qualitative project: details and dialogue. Sage, London

Morse J M 1991 Negotiating commitment and involvement in the nurse-patient relationship. Journal of Advanced Nursing 16:455-468

National Institute for Mental Health 2003 Recovery and change - mental health into the main stream. Department of Health, Leeds

NHS Executive 1996 24 hour nurse care for people with severe and enduring mental illness. NHS Executive, Leeds

NHS Executive Mental Health Task Force 1994 Work programme. Department of Health, London

Nolan P 1990 Psychiatric nursing - the first 100 years. Senior Nurse 10(10):20-23

Nolan P 1996 Science and the early development of mental health nursing. Nursing Standard 48(10):44-47

Office of National Statistics 1998 Social trensa. Stationary Office, London

Owen S, Sweeney J 1995 The future role of the mental health nurse. Nurse Education Today 15:17-21

Pearson P 1997 Integrating qualitative and quantitative data analysis. Nurse Researcher 4(3):69-80

Peplau H 1988 Interpersonal relations in nursing. Macmillan, Basingstoke

Peplau H 1994 Psychiatric mental health nursing: challenge and change. Journal of Psychiatric and Mental Health Nursing 1:3-7

Peterson A, Bunton R, Foucault 1997 Health and Medicine. Routledge, London

Repper J, Ford R, Cooke A 1994 How can nurses build trusting relationships with people who have severe and long-term mental health problems? Experiences of case managers and their clients. Journal of Advanced Nursing 19:1096-1104

Rogers A, Pilgrim D 1994 Service users views of psychiatric nurses. British Journal of Nursing 3(1):16-18

Rogers A, Pilgrim D 2001 Mental health policy in Britain. Palgrave, Basingstoke

Rolfe G 1994 Some factors associated with change in patient-centredness of student nurses during the common foundation programme in nursing. International Journal of Nursing Studies 31(5):421-436

Rudman M 1996 User involvement in mental health nursing practice: rhetoric or reality? Journal of Psychiatric and Mental Health Nursing 3(6):385-390

Sainsbury Centre for Mental Health 1998 Acute problems: a survey of the quality of care in acute psychiatric wards. The Sainsbury Centre for Mental Health, London

Sayce L 2000 From psychiatric patient to citizen: overcoming stigma and social exclusion. Macmillan, Basingstoke

Seccombe I, Smith G 1996 In the balance: registered nurse supply and demand - a summary. Institute of Employment Studies, University of Sussex, Brighton

Sheppard D 1996 Learning the lessons, 2nd edn. The Zito Trust, London

Silverman D 1997 Qualitative research: theory, method and practice. Sage, London

Smart B 1993 Postmodernity. Routledge, London

Social Services Inspectorate 1995 Social services departments and the care programme approach: an inspection. Department of Health, London

Tilley S 1997 The mental health nurse. Blackwell, London

Towell D 1975 Understanding psychiatric nursing. RCN, London

Tudor K 1996 Mental health promotion: paradigms and practice. Routledge, London

United Kingdom Central Council for Nursing, Midwifery and Health Visiting 1986 Project 2000 - a new preparation for practice. UKCC, London

United Kingdom Central Council for Nursing, Midwifery and Health Visiting 1987 Project 2000 - the final proposals. Project paper 9. UKCC, London

Welsh Institute for Health and Social Care 1998 Healthcare futures 2010. University of Glanmorgan, Pontypridd

White E, Riley E, Davis S, Twinn S 1994 A detailed study of the relationship between teaching, support, supervision and role modelling in clinical areas, within the context of the project 2000 courses. ENB, London

Index